INFUSION MASTERY

*The Ultimate Handbook Of Vital
Compounds In IV Hydration Therapy*

CATIE HARRIS,PHD, MBA, RN

CONTENTS

ABOUT THE AUTHOR

Catie Harris, PhD, RN, MBA is the owner and CEO of NursePreneurs. She started offering an IV Hydration course after multiple requests in her Facebook Community for support in this area. Catie partnered with nurses who already owned IV Hydration businesses to create a step by step program for nurses who wanted to get started in this business model. In putting together the program, the team found that there was a lack of information out there in regards to the role of vitamins, minerals, amino acids, coenzymes and peptides. Over the years, NursePreneurs has amassed a lot of information but it wasn't centralized in any one place, making it difficult to share this information. Therefore, it was decided to compile everything that was learned into this book. NursePreneurs is thrilled to bring to our community the ultimate handbook for IV therapies.

DISCLAIMER

The information provided in this text regarding IV hydration therapies is intended for educational purposes only and should not be considered medical advice. The content is not meant to replace the guidance, diagnosis, or treatment provided by healthcare professionals.

While we strive to ensure the accuracy and timeliness of the information presented, medical knowledge is constantly evolving, and new research may modify the understanding of certain concepts or treatments. Therefore, we cannot guarantee the completeness, accuracy, or reliability of the information provided.

Any reliance on the information presented in this text is solely at your own risk. We recommend consulting a qualified healthcare professional before making any decisions or taking any actions based on the information provided. Only a healthcare professional can properly assess your unique medical situation and provide appropriate advice or treatment.

The content in this text does not establish a doctor-patient relationship between the reader and the author or publisher. It is crucial to consult with a qualified healthcare professional for personalized medical advice related to your specific condition.

Furthermore, the mention of any specific products, services, or healthcare facilities in this text does not constitute an endorsement or recommendation by the author or publisher. The inclusion of such references is purely for informational purposes and should not be interpreted as a guarantee of their efficacy or safety.

In summary, this text on IV hydration therapies is intended for educational purposes only. It is not a substitute for professional medical advice, diagnosis, or treatment. Please consult a qualified healthcare professional for personalized medical guidance based on your specific circumstances.

FREE GIFT

NursePreneurs would like to give a special thanks to all our readership. We strive hard to improve all the time and bring the best of the best to our audience.

In addition to the contents of this book, NursePreneurs invites you to get our Quick Start Guide, our breakeven spreadsheet and our top formulas workbook for free.

SImply sign up here to get access: https://tinyurl.com/ivquickstart

CERTIFICATION

Learn more about our IV Hydration certification process at

https://NursePreneurs.com/certification

OVERVIEW

In today's fast-paced world, maintaining optimal health and well-being is of utmost importance. The rise in diagnosis of chronic diseases, stress, and poor nutrition has left many people searching for ways to improve their overall health and vitality. IV hydration therapy has emerged as a promising solution, offering individuals the opportunity to replenish essential nutrients, vitamins, and minerals that may be lacking in their daily lives. This book, *IV Hydration Therapy*, provides a comprehensive guide on this revolutionary treatment and how it can benefit a wide range of conditions.

IV hydration therapy involves the administration of nutrients, vitamins, minerals, amino acids, and other essential substances directly into the bloodstream through intravenous infusion. By bypassing the digestive system, these vital components can be delivered more efficiently and effectively to the body's cells, tissues, and organs. IV infusion's goal is to maximize absorption and utilization of nutrients, allowing individuals to experience rapid and lasting benefits.

The benefits of IV hydration therapy are numerous, and it is useful for a variety of health conditions and bodily symptoms. In this book, we will explore 25 conditions and general areas that can benefit from IV hydration therapy, including but not limited to:

1. Fatigue

2. Dehydration

3. Migraines

4. Hangovers

5. Nutrient deficiencies

6. Chronic pain

7. Fibromyalgia

8. Chronic fatigue syndrome

9. Cold and flu symptoms

10. Athletic performance and recovery

11. Jet lag

12. Skin health and anti-aging

13. Detoxification

14. Weight loss

15. Anxiety and stress management

16. Immune system support

17. Asthma and allergies

18. Autoimmune disorders

19. Inflammatory conditions

20. Cognitive function and memory

21. Mood disorders

22. Cancer treatment support

23. Wound healing

24. Anemia

25. Gastrointestinal disorders

Throughout this book, we will delve into the essential components of IV hydration therapy including vitamins, minerals, amino acids, coenzymes, nutrients, and more. Understanding the functions and benefits of each element will enable you to make informed decisions about the best course of action for your unique needs and those of the clients you serve.

We will also provide detailed discussion of protocols and treatment plans, offering practical guidance on how to safely and effectively implement IV hydration therapy into healthcare regimens. From dosages and administration to contraindications and precautions, this book will equip you with the necessary knowledge to optimize your IV hydration therapy offerings.

The information provided in *IV Hydration Therapy* is crucial for anyone interested in enhancing health and well-being. Whether you are a healthcare professional, a patient seeking alternative treatments, or simply curious about this innovative approach, this book will serve as a valuable resource in the journey towards optimal health.

IV hydration therapy has the potential to transform lives by addressing a wide array of health concerns and improving overall wellness. With the knowledge gained from this book, you will be well-equipped to harness the power of IV hydration therapy and unlock the door to a healthier life for you, your clients, or whomever you seek to serve.

CHAPTER 1 - HOW TO USE THIS BOOK

For years, NursePreneurs has been running its IV Hydration program with a focus on formulas. It became obvious from repeated student and customer questions that the specific functionality of each ingredient drew curiosity at a minimum, if not full blown skepticism. There are certainly numerous textbooks that detail the chemical composition and arrangement of the molecules, but data and information clinically relevant to IV hydration therapy seems to be scarce. Equally problematic is the overall lack of research interest in this area. While there is extensive research on individual vitamins, minerals and amino acids, most of it needs to be extrapolated and applied to IV Hydration.

With all of that in mind, we decided that an IV hydration clinical handbook would be best designed as a breakdown of clinically relevant information that both supports the operation of an IV hydration clinic and provides useful guidance on explaining the "what and why" of various formula ingredients to your laymen clients. Let's be honest - most people do not need to know the nitty gritty of things like stereoisomers. They just want to know how a particular ingredient is going to help them.

Please note that while we have made recommendations regarding IV hydration administration quantities and delivery frequencies, they are made solely based on scientific evidence rather than clinical data.

From our extensive literature search, we have not been able to locate any standardized or universally accepted IV hydration formulas.

Your formulas and IV hydration packages, whether borrowed from colleagues or uniquely your own, should be reviewed and approved by your medical director. Of course, they should also always be developed with the best interest of the client in mind. This book is a general educational resource only. This book does not offer patient-specific medical advice and does not replace the guidance or advice of an individual's qualified medical provider nor that of a business's medical director.

CHAPTER 2 - WHAT YOU NEED TO KNOW

Vitamins and minerals are both essential nutrients that are required in small amounts for the proper functioning of the body. However, there are some key differences between the two:

1. Chemical structure: Vitamins are organic compounds, which means they contain carbon and are produced by living organisms. Minerals, on the other hand, are inorganic compounds, which means they do not contain carbon and are naturally occurring.

2. Required amounts: Vitamins are required in small amounts and are classified as either fat-soluble (vitamins A, D, E, and K) or water-soluble (vitamins B and C). Fat-soluble vitamins can be stored in the body, whereas water-soluble vitamins are not stored and must be consumed regularly. Minerals are also required in small amounts, but are not classified as fat-soluble or water-soluble.

3. Function: Vitamins and minerals have different functions in the body. Vitamins are involved in various processes, such as energy production, immune function, and cell growth and development. Minerals are involved in processes such as muscle and nerve function, bone health, and the formation of red blood cells.

4. Sources: Vitamins and minerals can be obtained from food and supplements. Vitamins are primarily found in plant and

animal-based foods, whereas minerals are found in soil and water, and are absorbed by plants and animals.

It is important to consume adequate amounts of both vitamins and minerals in order to maintain good health. A balanced diet that includes a variety of nutrient-rich foods can help ensure that you are getting all the vitamins and minerals your body needs. If you are concerned about your nutrient intake, it is important to speak with a healthcare provider or registered dietitian.

Amino acids are the building blocks of proteins, and they play many important roles in the body, including supporting muscle growth and repair, promoting immune function, and providing energy. In IV hydration clinics, amino acids are often used to help replenish and nourish the body, particularly in cases of dehydration, malnutrition, or other conditions that affect protein metabolism.

Vitamins, minerals, and amino acids are essential nutrients that are required by the body for various physiological functions. Vitamins are organic compounds that the body needs in small quantities to maintain normal metabolism, growth, and development. There are 13 essential vitamins, and each has a unique role in the body. For example, Vitamin A helps with vision, immune function, and skin health, while Vitamin C is an antioxidant that helps with immune function and collagen synthesis. B vitamins are a group of vitamins that help the body convert food into energy, support nervous system function, and promote overall wellness.

Minerals are inorganic compounds that the body needs for various functions such as building strong bones, maintaining fluid balance, and producing energy. There are two types of minerals: macrominerals and trace minerals. Macrominerals are required in larger quantities, while trace minerals are needed in smaller amounts. Examples of major minerals include calcium, magnesium, and sodium, while trace minerals include iron, zinc, and copper.

In IV hydration therapy, vitamins, minerals, and amino acids may be used to help replenish and nourish the body, particularly in cases of dehydration, malnutrition, or other conditions that affect nutrient absorption or metabolism. IV therapy allows for the delivery of nutrients directly into the bloodstream, bypassing the digestive system and ensuring that the nutrients are absorbed quickly and efficiently.

The specific vitamins, minerals, and amino acids used in IV hydration therapy may vary depending on the individual needs of the patient and the goals of the treatment. For example, IV Vitamin C may be used to boost the immune system, while a combination of B vitamins may be used to improve energy levels and support nervous system function. IV amino acids such as glutamine and arginine may be used to support recovery after surgery or illness.

Vitamins, minerals, and amino acids that are commonly used in IV hydration therapy include:

1. Vitamin C: A powerful antioxidant that supports immune function and helps fight inflammation.

2. B vitamins (B1, B2, B3, B5, B6, and B12): Important for energy production and metabolism, and help maintain healthy skin, hair, and eyes.

3. Magnesium: An essential mineral that helps regulate muscle and nerve function, and plays a role in the immune system.

4. Calcium: Important for healthy bones, muscle function, and nerve function.

5. Zinc: Helps support the immune system, and is involved in wound healing and DNA synthesis.

6. Selenium: An antioxidant that supports immune function, and is important for thyroid health.

7. Glutathione: A powerful antioxidant that helps protect cells from damage, and plays a role in detoxification.

8. Amino acids (e.g., arginine, lysine, cysteine): Building blocks of protein that are important for muscle growth and repair, immune function, and other bodily processes.

There are some vitamins, minerals, and amino acids that are not commonly used in IV hydration therapy due to their potential side effects. For example, high doses of vitamin A can be toxic, and high doses of iron can cause nausea, vomiting, and other gastrointestinal symptoms.

Additionally, certain amino acids (e.g., methionine) may not be appropriate for individuals with certain medical conditions. It is important for healthcare providers to carefully evaluate a patient's medical history and overall health before recommending IV hydration therapy and to use appropriate dosages and combinations of nutrients.

CHAPTER 3 - VITAMINS

Vitamins are organic compounds that play crucial roles in various biochemical processes in the human body. These essential micronutrients cannot be synthesized by the body in sufficient amounts and must be obtained through diet or supplementation. Vitamins are vital for maintaining overall health, growth, and development. They function as coenzymes, antioxidants, and precursors for other essential molecules in the body.

VITAMIN CLASSIFICATION

Vitamins are classified into two groups: fat-soluble and water-soluble. Fat-soluble vitamins include vitamins A, D, E, and K, while water-soluble vitamins include the B complex vitamins and vitamin C.

Fat-soluble vitamins:

Fat-soluble vitamins are absorbed in the body along with dietary fats, then are stored in the liver and adipose tissues. They tend to have a longer half-life in the body compared to water-soluble vitamins, which means they can accumulate and potentially reach toxic levels if consumed in excessive amounts.

A. Vitamin A (Retinol): This vitamin is essential for vision, immune system function, growth and development, and the maintenance of epithelial tissues. It is found in animal-based foods such as liver, dairy products, and fish oils, as well as plant-based sources like carrots, sweet potatoes, and leafy greens in the form of provitamin A (beta-carotene).

B. Vitamin D (Cholecalciferol): Vitamin D is synthesized in the skin upon exposure to sunlight and is also found in foods such as fatty fish, fortified milk, and egg yolks. It plays a vital role in calcium and phosphorus homeostasis, bone health, and immune function.

C. Vitamin E (Tocopherol): This vitamin acts as an antioxidant, protecting cell membranes and lipids from oxidative damage. It is found in vegetable oils, nuts, seeds, and leafy green vegetables.

D. Vitamin K (Phylloquinone and Menaquinone): Vitamin K is necessary for blood clotting and bone metabolism. It is found in green leafy vegetables, fermented foods, and some animal products.

Water-soluble vitamins: Water-soluble vitamins are not stored in the body, and excess amounts are excreted in urine. This means that they need to be consumed regularly to maintain adequate levels. The B complex vitamins and vitamin C fall into this category.

A. Vitamin B Complex: The B complex vitamins are a group of eight water-soluble vitamins that play critical roles in energy production, brain function, and metabolism. They include B1 (thiamine), B2 (riboflavin), B3 (niacin), B5 (pantothenic acid), B6 (pyridoxine), B7 (biotin), B9 (folic acid), and B12 (cobalamin).

B. Vitamin C (Ascorbic acid): This water-soluble vitamin is a powerful antioxidant, helps with collagen synthesis, and is vital for immune function. It is found in fruits and vegetables, particularly citrus fruits, berries, kiwi, and bell peppers.

VITAMIN FUNCTIONS

Vitamins participate in a wide range of physiological processes in the body. They act as coenzymes, assisting enzymes in catalyzing chemical reactions. For instance, many B vitamins function as coenzymes in essential metabolic pathways, such as energy production, amino acid metabolism, and the synthesis of nucleic acids.

Some vitamins also function as antioxidants, neutralizing harmful free radicals that can cause cellular damage. Vitamin C, for example, is a potent antioxidant that protects cells from oxidative stress, supports the immune system, and aids in the synthesis of collagen, a protein necessary for healthy skin, blood vessels, and connective tissues.

Vitamins also play roles in hormone synthesis and regulation, immune function, and gene expression. For example, vitamin D acts as a hormone that regulates calcium and phosphorus levels in the body, maintaining bone health and preventing conditions like rickets and osteoporosis. Vitamin A is essential for maintaining the integrity of epithelial tissues and plays a critical role in vision and immune function.

VITAMIN DEFICIENCIES AND TOXICITIES

Inadequate intake of vitamins can lead to deficiencies that may manifest as a variety of health problems. Some common vitamin deficiencies include:

1. Vitamin A deficiency: It can lead to night blindness, impaired immune function, and skin problems.

2. Vitamin D deficiency: It can result in rickets in children and osteomalacia or osteoporosis in adults.

3. Vitamin B12 deficiency: It can cause megaloblastic anemia, peripheral neuropathy, and cognitive dysfunction.

On the other hand, excessive intake of certain vitamins can result in toxicities. For example, hypervitaminosis A can lead to nausea, vomiting, hair loss, and even liver damage, while hypervitaminosis D can cause hypercalcemia, leading to kidney stones, calcification of soft tissues, and kidney damage. It is essential to maintain a balanced intake of vitamins to avoid both deficiencies and toxicities.

VITAMIN SOURCES AND SUPPLEMENTATION

A well-balanced diet that includes a variety of fruits, vegetables, whole grains, lean proteins, and healthy fats should provide adequate amounts of vitamins to maintain overall health. However, certain populations may be at risk for vitamin deficiencies due to factors such as age, pregnancy, medical conditions, or dietary restrictions.

In such cases, vitamin supplementation may be necessary to ensure adequate intake. Supplementation should be done under the guidance of a healthcare professional, who can determine the appropriate dosage and duration based on individual needs.

We know that vitamins are essential micronutrients that play crucial roles in maintaining overall health and supporting various physiological processes. We know that a well-balanced diet is the key to obtaining adequate amounts of these vital compounds. However, certain individuals may require supplementation to meet their specific needs. It is crucial to understand the functions, sources, and potential deficiencies or toxicities associated with vitamins to maintain optimal health and well-being.

For the rest of this chapter, we will provide in-depth information on the vitamins used in IV Hydration. Please note fat-soluble vitamins are not typically used in IV therapy for a variety of reasons including the theoretical risk of a fat embolus. Vitamin D is included in this list but is given as an IM shot and not in an IV bag. Vitamins A, E, and K will not be discussed.

VITAMIN C

Vitamin C, also known as ascorbic acid, is a water-soluble vitamin and a powerful antioxidant. It plays several important roles in the body, including:

- Collagen production: Vitamin C is essential for the synthesis of collagen, a protein that provides structure and support to connective tissues, skin, bones, and blood vessels.

- Immune function: It strengthens the immune system by enhancing the function of immune cells and supporting the production of antibodies.

- Wound healing: Vitamin C helps repair damaged tissues and promotes faster wound healing.

- Iron absorption: It increases the absorption of non-heme iron from plant-based sources, preventing iron deficiency anemia.

- Antioxidant protection: Vitamin C neutralizes harmful free radicals, reducing oxidative stress and preventing cellular damage.

Dosage Recommendations

The Recommended Dietary Allowance (RDA) for vitamin C varies depending on age, sex, and life stage. Here are the general guidelines for daily vitamin C intake:

- Adult men: 90 mg

- Adult women: 75 mg

- Pregnant women: 85 mg

- Breastfeeding women: 120 mg

- Smokers: Add an additional 35 mg to the RDA for your sex and life stage

For IV hydration, the dosage of vitamin C can range from 500 mg to 15,000 mg, depending on the patient's needs and medical conditions. High-dose vitamin C infusions (above 15,000 mg) may be used to treat specific conditions under medical supervision.

Conditions Treated with Vitamin C

Vitamin C infusions can be used to treat or prevent several conditions, including:

- Vitamin C deficiency (scurvy)

- Fatigue

- Common cold

- Iron deficiency anemia (by improving iron absorption)

- Skin aging and wrinkles (by promoting collagen production)

- Oxidative stress-related conditions

- High-dose vitamin C IV infusions, such as 15gm+ (15-100gm),are typically administered for specific medical conditions or in certain clinical situations. Blood work, such as a complete blood count (CBC) and kidney function tests, may be required before starting high-dose vitamin C therapy. Some instances when high-dose vitamin C might be considered include:

- Cancer treatment support: Some studies suggest that high-dose vitamin C, when administered intravenously, may help improve the quality of life of cancer patients, reduce chemotherapy side effects, and potentially slow down the progression of certain types of cancer. However, more research is needed to establish the efficacy and safety of high-dose vitamin C as a cancer treatment adjunct.

- Chronic viral infections: High-dose vitamin C infusions have been used to support the immune system in cases of chronic viral infections, such as Epstein-Barr virus, cytomegalovirus, or human herpesvirus 6. The idea is to enhance the body's natural defenses against these viruses, but more research is required to validate this approach.

- Chronic fatigue syndrome (CFS) and fibromyalgia: Some practitioners have used high-dose vitamin C infusions to help manage symptoms of CFS and fibromyalgia, including fatigue, muscle pain, and cognitive dysfunction. However, the effectiveness of this treatment for these conditions remains inconclusive, and more research is needed.

- Oxidative stress-related conditions: High-dose vitamin C infusions might be beneficial in situations where the body experiences high levels of oxidative stress, such as severe infections or inflammatory conditions. As a powerful antioxidant, vitamin C can help neutralize harmful free radicals and reduce oxidative stress in the body.

Signs of Vitamin C Deficiency

Vitamin C deficiency is rare in developed countries but can occur in individuals with limited access to fresh fruits and vegetables. Signs of deficiency include:

- Fatigue

- Muscle weakness

- Joint and muscle aches

- Swollen, bleeding gums

- Bruising easily

- Dry, scaly skin

- Slow wound healing

Signs of Vitamin C Toxicity

Vitamin C toxicity is unlikely due to its water-soluble nature, but excessive intake (above 2,000 mg per day) can cause side effects, such as:

- Diarrhea

- Nausea

- Abdominal cramps

- Headaches

- Insomnia

- Kidney stones (in susceptible individuals)

Contraindications

IV vitamin C infusions should be used with caution or avoided in the following situations:

- History of kidney stones or kidney disease

- Hemochromatosis (iron overload disorder)

- Glucose-6-phosphate dehydrogenase (G6PD) deficiency

- Pregnancy and breastfeeding (consult with a healthcare provider)

What People Say About Getting This Infusion

Anecdotal stories suggest that high-dose vitamin C infusions can help cancer patients by improving their quality of life, reducing side effects of chemotherapy, and enhancing their overall well-being. Some patients have reported increased energy levels, improved mood, and better immune function after receiving high-dose vitamin C infusions. However, it's essential to keep in mind that these stories are anecdotal, and more scientific research is needed to confirm the efficacy of high-dose vitamin C for cancer treatment.

Reasons to Promote Vitamin C

As a powerful antioxidant, Vitamin C plays a crucial role in collagen production – the protein responsible for maintaining your skin's elasticity and youthful appearance. As we age, our collagen production naturally declines, leading to the formation of wrinkles, fine lines, and sagging skin.

That's where IV Vitamin C therapy comes in. By delivering a potent dose of Vitamin C directly into your bloodstream, we bypass any absorption barriers associated with oral supplementation. Our IV therapy ensures that you receive the full benefits of Vitamin C, which include:

- Stimulating collagen production for firmer, smoother, and more radiant skin

- Reducing the appearance of wrinkles and fine lines

- Protecting your skin from oxidative stress and environmental damage

- Boosting your overall skin health and vitality

Treatment Protocol Suggestions

(Please note that there is no evidence-based literature to support treatment protocols to date. You will need to discuss with your medical director to determine the final protocols. These are for educational purposes only.)

1. Cold and Flu: During the initial phase, IV vitamin C treatments may be given once per day for the first 2-3 days. This frequency helps to provide a concentrated boost of vitamin C to support the immune system and reduce the severity and duration of symptoms. After the initial phase, the frequency of treatments can be reduced. Recovery treatments may be given once every 1-2 days for an additional 3-5 days, depending on the individual's response to the therapy. Example: Vitamin C 5gm daily x 3 days

2. Cancer treatment support: High-dose IV vitamin C may be given 2-3 times per week, depending on the patient's tolerance. Example: 50gm 2x per week x 3 months

3. Chronic fatigue syndrome (CFS) or fibromyalgia: Treatments may be given 1-2 times per week for several weeks, followed by a maintenance phase of once every 2-4 weeks, depending

on the patient's response. Example: 15gm 1x/week x 1 month, then 1x/month ongoing

4. Chronic viral infections: High-dose IV vitamin C may be given 1-3 times per week, depending on the patient's condition. Example: 15gm 2x/week x 3 months

5. Oxidative Stress: The frequency of IV vitamin C treatments for oxidative stress-related conditions can vary. In some cases, treatments may be given once or twice per week for several weeks, followed by a maintenance phase of once every 2-4 weeks. The treatment frequency will depend on the patient's response to the therapy. Example: 15gm 2x/week for 1 month, then once per month.

6. Skin Conditions: Initial Phase: During the initial phase, IV vitamin C treatments may be given once or twice per week for 4 to 6 weeks. This frequency helps to provide a concentrated boost of vitamin C to promote collagen production, reduce inflammation, and improve the overall appearance of the skin. Maintenance Phase: After the initial phase, the frequency of treatments can be reduced to a maintenance schedule. Maintenance treatments may be given once every 2-4 weeks, depending on the individual's response to the therapy and the healthcare provider's recommendation. Example: 5gm 2x/week for 6 weeks, then once per month.

Clinical Information

1. What forms does vitamin C come in?
Vitamin C is available in various forms, including tablets, capsules, chewables, powders, and liquids.

2. What are the daily dosage limits?

   The recommended daily allowance (RDA) for vitamin C varies depending on age, sex, and other factors. For adults, the RDA for vitamin C is typically 75-90 milligrams per day. However, higher doses of vitamin C, up to 2000 milligrams per day, may be used for certain conditions under medical supervision.

3. How is vitamin C stored?

   Vitamin C is a relatively unstable compound that is sensitive to heat, light, and air. Vitamin C supplements should be stored in a cool, dry place, away from direct sunlight and heat. Liquid vitamin C supplements should be refrigerated after opening.

4. How is vitamin C prepared for IV infusion?

   Vitamin C can be prepared for IV infusion by reconstituting it with sterile water or saline solution. The prepared solution should be used immediately or refrigerated for later use. It is important to use freshly prepared vitamin C solutions for IV infusion to ensure maximal potency and efficacy.

5. Treatment protocols:

   Vitamin C has been studied for its potential therapeutic benefits in various health conditions, including cancer, infections, and cardiovascular disease. However, the optimal dosage and duration of vitamin C supplementation for different health conditions have not been fully established and may vary depending on the individual's needs and response to treatment. For example, for the treatment of sepsis, a protocol may involve high-dose IV vitamin C (up to 6 grams per day) for several days. For the treatment of cancer, vitamin C may be used in combination with other therapies, and dosages may range from 1 to 100 grams per day.

6. What is the half-life of vitamin C?

   The half-life of vitamin C in the body is relatively short - approximately 30 minutes to 2 hours. This short half-life means that vitamin C levels can quickly decrease after supplementation is discontinued.

7. Is it stable?

   Vitamin C is a relatively unstable compound that is sensitive to heat, light, and air. Vitamin C supplements should be stored in a cool, dry place, away from direct sunlight and heat. Liquid vitamin C supplements should be refrigerated after opening. Be careful not to inject any air into the vial.

References

1. Carr, A. C., & Maggini, S. (2017). Vitamin C and immune function. Nutrients, 9(11), 1211.

2. Chambial, S., Dwivedi, S., Shukla, K. K., John, P. J., & Sharma, P. (2013). Vitamin C in disease prevention and cure: an overview. Indian Journal of Clinical Biochemistry, 28(4), 314-328.

3. Pullar, J. M., Carr, A. C., & Vissers, M. C. (2017). The roles of vitamin C in skin health. Nutrients, 9(8), 866.

4. Schleicher, R. L., Carroll, M. D., Ford, E. S., & Lacher, D. A. (2009). Serum vitamin C and the prevalence of vitamin C deficiency in the United States: 2003-2004 National Health and Nutrition Examination Survey (NHANES). The American journal of clinical nutrition, 90(5), 1252-1263.

5. Padayatty, S. J., Sun, H., Wang, Y., Riordan, H. D., Hewitt, S. M., Katz, A., ... & Levine, M. (2004). Vitamin C pharmacokinetics: implications for oral and intravenous use. Annals of internal medicine, 140(7), 533-537.

VITAMIN B COMPLEX

Vitamin B Complex is a powerful group of vitamins. We will explore each of these vitamins individually, but here are some overall benefits of supplementing with the Bs.

1. Increased energy: The B vitamins, especially B12 and B6, play a crucial role in converting food into energy. IV vitamin B complex can help provide a quick boost of energy for those who are feeling fatigued or run down.

2. Improved immune function: B vitamins are essential for a healthy immune system. IV vitamin B complex can help support the body's natural defense mechanisms and reduce the risk of infections and illness.

3. Enhanced cognitive function: Several of the B vitamins, including B6, B12, and folate, are important for brain

function and development. IV vitamin B complex may help improve memory, focus, and overall cognitive function.

4. Reduced stress and anxiety: B vitamins are known to play a role in reducing stress and anxiety levels. IV vitamin B complex can help provide a calming effect and may reduce the symptoms of anxiety and depression.

5. Better skin, hair, and nails: B vitamins are important for healthy skin, hair, and nails. IV vitamin B complex can help improve the appearance and texture of these features.

6. Improved cardiovascular health: Some studies suggest that IV vitamin B complex may help reduce the risk of heart disease by lowering levels of homocysteine, an amino acid that can contribute to heart disease.

Reasons To Promote B Complex

1. Energy: The B vitamins are essential for energy production, helping to convert food into fuel for the body. They also help to support the function of the adrenal glands, which play a crucial role in stress response and energy regulation.

2. Nerve function: The B vitamins are important for the maintenance of healthy nerve function, helping to transmit signals between the brain and body.

3. Cell growth and repair: The B vitamins play a key role in DNA synthesis and cell division, helping to support the growth and repair of tissues throughout the body.

4. Skin health: Several of the B vitamins, including biotin and niacin, are important for maintaining healthy skin, hair, and nails.

5. Mood regulation: Vitamin B12 and folate are important for mood regulation and may help to prevent or alleviate symptoms of depression and anxiety.

Treatment Protocol Suggestions

(Please note that there is no evidence-basedevidence-d based literature to support any treatment protocols to date. You will need to discuss with your medical director to determine the final protocols. These are for educational purposes only.).

For all conditions, clients may benefit from more frequent infusions initially followed by maintenance therapy. Example: Vitamin B Complex infusion 1x/week for 1 month then once a month ongoing. Consider pairing this drip with adjuvant therapies such as infrared light.

VITAMIN B1 (THIAMINE)

Vitamin B1, also known as thiamine, is a water-soluble vitamin that plays a crucial role in energy metabolism, nerve function, and brain health. As nurses interested in starting an IV hydration clinic, it is essential to understand the benefits, dosage recommendations, conditions treated, signs of deficiency and toxicity, contraindications, and other relevant information about this vital nutrient.

Benefits of Vitamin B1

1. Energy metabolism: Thiamine helps convert carbohydrates into energy, supporting cellular function and overall health.

2. Nerve function: Thiamine is essential for the proper functioning of the nervous system, as it plays a role in the production of neurotransmitters and the maintenance of myelin sheaths.

3. Brain health: Thiamine supports cognitive function and memory, and has been used to treat certain neurological disorders, such as Wernicke-Korsakoff syndrome.

Dosage Recommendations

The Recommended Dietary Allowance (RDA) for thiamine is 1.2 mg/day for adult males and 1.1 mg/day for adult females. In an IV hydration setting, thiamine dosages may vary depending on the specific formulation and individual needs. Consultation with a healthcare professional is necessary to determine the appropriate dosage for each patient.

Conditions Treated with Vitamin B1

1. Thiamine deficiency (beriberi): Thiamine is used to treat beriberi, a condition characterized by muscle weakness, peripheral neuropathy, and heart failure.

2. Wernicke-Korsakoff syndrome: Thiamine is essential for the treatment of this neurological disorder, often associated with

chronic alcoholism, which can cause confusion, memory loss, and ataxia.

3. Other neurological disorders: Thiamine may be used as part of the treatment for conditions such as Alzheimer's disease, multiple sclerosis, and peripheral neuropathy.

Signs of Vitamin B1 Deficiency

1. Fatigue and weakness

2. Muscle wasting and atrophy

3. Peripheral neuropathy (tingling, numbness, or pain in the extremities)

4. Swelling (edema)

5. Confusion, memory loss, or cognitive decline

Signs of Vitamin B1 Toxicity

Thiamine toxicity is rare, as the body can efficiently excrete excess amounts through urine. However, very high doses may cause adverse effects such as:

1. Headaches

2. Nausea and vomiting

3. Skin rashes

4. Hypersensitivity reactions

Contraindications

Thiamine should be used with caution in patients with a known hypersensitivity to the vitamin or any component of the infusion formulation. Additionally, thiamine should be administered with care in patients with severe liver or kidney dysfunction.

Special Notes

In addition to treating thiamine deficiency and related neurological disorders, thiamine has also been used as an adjunct therapy in certain conditions, such as diabetic neuropathy, congestive heart failure, and inflammatory bowel disease. Bariatric surgery, such as gastric bypass or sleeve gastrectomy, can lead to nutrient deficiencies due to reduced food intake and altered nutrient absorption. Thiamine deficiency is one such possible outcome. Consider working with Bariatric surgeons to supplement required thiamine stores.

Frequency of Treatments

The frequency of thiamine treatments in an IV hydration setting will depend on the individual patient's needs and the specific condition being treated. Typically, hiamine is part of a vitamin B complex treatment and not given alone.

Clinical Information

1. What forms does vitamin B1 come in?
   Vitamin B1 is available in various forms, including capsules, tablets, injections, and IV infusions.

2. What are the daily dosage limits?

   The recommended daily dosage of vitamin B1 varies depending on age, gender, and health status. For adults, the recommended daily allowance (RDA) of vitamin B1 is 1.1-1.2 mg per day, with higher doses recommended for pregnant and lactating women.

3. How is vitamin B1 stored?

   Vitamin B1 should be stored in a cool, dry place, away from direct sunlight and heat, to ensure maximal potency and efficacy.

4. How is vitamin B1 prepared for IV infusion?

   Vitamin B1 can be prepared for IV infusion by diluting it with sterile water or saline solution. The prepared solution should be used immediately or refrigerated for later use. It is important to use freshly prepared vitamin B1 solutions for IV infusion to ensure maximal potency and efficacy.

5. Treatment protocols:

   Vitamin B1 is used to treat or prevent thiamine deficiency, a condition that can occur in individuals who consume a diet low in thiamine or who have difficulty absorbing thiamine from their diet. Thiamine deficiency can lead to a range of symptoms, including weakness, fatigue, muscle pain, and neuropathy. Intravenous (IV) administration of thiamine may be used to treat severe cases of thiamine deficiency or to rapidly restore thiamine levels in individuals who are unable to absorb oral thiamine supplements. The recommended dosage and duration of IV thiamine therapy depend on the severity of the deficiency and the individual's response to treatment.

6. What is the half-life of vitamin B1?
   The half-life of vitamin B1 in the body is relatively short - approximately 2 hours. This means that thiamine levels in the body can quickly decline if a continuous supply of thiamine is not provided.

7. Is it stable?
   Vitamin B1 is a relatively stable compound that is not affected by heat or light. However, thiamine can be rapidly degraded in the presence of oxygen or in alkaline environments. Vitamin B1 supplements should be stored in a cool, dry place, away from direct sunlight and heat, to ensure maximal potency and efficacy.

References

1. Lonsdale, D. (2006). A review of the biochemistry, metabolism and clinical benefits of thiamin(e) and its derivatives. Evidence-Based Complementary and Alternative Medicine, 3(1), 49-59.

2. National Institutes of Health, Office of Dietary Supplements. (2021). Thiamin: Fact Sheet for Health Professionals. Retrieved from https://ods.od.nih.gov/factsheets/Thiamin-HealthProfessional/

3. Subramanya, S. B., & Subramanian, V. S. (2020). Vitamin B1 (thiamine) and dementia. Annals of the New York Academy of Sciences, 1467(1), 21-29.

4. World Health Organization. (1999). Thiamine deficiency and its prevention and control in major emergencies. Retrieved from https://www.who.int/publications/i/item/WHO-NHD-99.13

VITAMIN B2 (RIBOFLAVIN)

Vitamin B2, also known as riboflavin, is a water-soluble vitamin that plays a critical role in energy production, cellular function, and the maintenance of skin and eye health. It is crucial to understand the benefits, dosage recommendations, conditions treated, signs of deficiency and toxicity, contraindications, and other relevant information about this essential nutrient.

Benefits of Vitamin B2

1. Energy production: Riboflavin is a key component in the formation of flavin coenzymes (FAD and FMN), which participate in essential metabolic processes, including the production of energy from carbohydrates, fats, and proteins.

2. Cellular function: Riboflavin supports cellular growth, reproduction, and the maintenance of the body's antioxidant defenses.

3. Skin and eye health: Riboflavin is necessary for maintaining healthy skin, hair, and nails, as well as promoting good vision and protecting the eyes from oxidative stress.

Dosage Recommendations

The Recommended Dietary Allowance (RDA) for riboflavin is 1.3 mg/day for adult males and 1.1 mg/day for adult females. In an IV hydration setting, riboflavin dosages may vary depending on the specific formulation and individual needs. Consultation with a healthcare professional is necessary to determine the appropriate dosage for each patient.

Conditions Treated with Vitamin B2

1. Riboflavin deficiency (ariboflavinosis): Riboflavin is used to treat ariboflavinosis, a condition characterized by skin and mucous membrane lesions, anemia, and neurological symptoms.

2. Migraines: Riboflavin supplementation has been shown to help reduce the frequency and severity of migraines in some individuals.

3. Eye disorders: Riboflavin has been used in the treatment of certain eye conditions, such as cataracts and corneal disorders.

Signs of Vitamin B2 Deficiency

1. Cracked and red lips (cheilosis)

2. Inflammation and soreness of the mouth and tongue (stomatitis and glossitis)

3. Scaly, greasy skin rashes (seborrheic dermatitis)

4. Anemia

5. Sensitivity to light (photophobia) and eye fatigue

Signs of Vitamin B2 Toxicity

Riboflavin toxicity is rare, as excess amounts are efficiently excreted through urine. There are no known toxic effects associated with high riboflavin intake from food or supplements. However, extremely high doses may cause bright yellow-orange urine discoloration, which is generally harmless.

Contraindications

There are no known contraindications for riboflavin supplementation in an IV hydration setting. However, patients with a known hypersensitivity to riboflavin or any component of the infusion formulation should exercise caution.

Special Notes

In addition to treating riboflavin deficiency and migraines, riboflavin may also be used as an adjunct therapy for conditions such as:

1. Anemia: Riboflavin helps improve iron absorption and utilization, potentially benefiting those with iron-deficiency anemia.

2. Oxidative stress: Riboflavin's role in the body's antioxidant defenses may be beneficial in reducing oxidative stress related to various health conditions.

3. *Frequency of Treatments*

The frequency of riboflavin treatments in an IV hydration setting will depend on the individual patient's needs and the specific condition being treated. Typically riboflavin is part of a vitamin B Complex treatment and not given alone.

Clinical Information

1. What forms does vitamin B2 come in?
    Vitamin B2 (riboflavin) is available in various forms, including capsules, tablets, and liquids.

2. What are the daily dosage limits?
    The recommended daily allowance (RDA) for riboflavin is 1.1-1.3 mg for adults. However, higher doses may be necessary for individuals with certain health conditions or for therapeutic purposes.

3. How is vitamin B2 stored?
    Vitamin B2 supplements should be stored in a cool, dry place, away from direct sunlight and heat.

4. How is vitamin B2 prepared for IV infusion?
    Riboflavin can be prepared for IV infusion by diluting it with sterile water or saline solution. The prepared solution should be used immediately or refrigerated for later use. It is important to use freshly prepared riboflavin solutions for IV infusion to ensure maximal potency and efficacy.

5. Treatment protocols:

   Riboflavin is commonly used for the prevention and treatment of riboflavin deficiency, as well as for migraine headaches. For the treatment of migraines, a protocol may involve daily doses of 400 mg of riboflavin for up to 3 months.

6. What is the half-life of vitamin B2?

   The half-life of riboflavin in the body is relatively short-approximately 66-84 minutes.

7. Is it stable?

   Riboflavin is a relatively stable compound that is not affected by heat or light. It is sensitive to alkaline conditions and can be rapidly degraded in the presence of alkaline substances. Riboflavin supplements should be stored in a cool, dry place, away from direct sunlight and heat, to ensure maximal potency and efficacy.

References

1. Powers, H. J. (2003). Riboflavin (vitamin B-2) and health. The American Journal of Clinical Nutrition, 77(6), 1352-1360.

2. National Institutes of Health, Office of Dietary Supplements. (2021). Riboflavin: Fact Sheet for Health Professionals. Retrieved from https://ods.od.nih.gov/factsheets/Riboflavin-HealthProfessional/

3. Boehnke, C., Reuter, U., Flach, U., Schuh-Hofer, S., Einhäupl, K. M., & Arnold, G. (2004). High-dose riboflavin treatment is efficacious in migraine prophylaxis: an open study in a tertiary care centre. European Journal of Neurology, 11(7), 475-477.

VITAMIN B3 (NIACIN)

Vitamin B3, also known as niacin, is a water-soluble vitamin that plays a critical role in energy metabolism, cellular function, and the maintenance of skin, nerve, and digestive health.

Benefits of Vitamin B3

1. Energy metabolism: Niacin is a key component in the formation of nicotinamide adenine dinucleotide (NAD) and its phosphate form (NADP), which are essential coenzymes involved in various metabolic processes, including the production of energy from carbohydrates, fats, and proteins.

2. Cellular function: Niacin supports cellular growth, reproduction, and DNA repair.

3. Skin, nerve, and digestive health: Niacin is necessary for maintaining healthy skin, proper nerve function, and a well-functioning digestive system.

Dosage Recommendations

The Recommended Dietary Allowance (RDA) for niacin is 16 mg/day for adult males and 14 mg/day for adult females, expressed as niacin equivalents (NE). In an IV hydration setting, niacin doses may vary depending on the specific formulation and individual needs. Consultation with a healthcare professional is necessary to determine the appropriate dosage for each patient.

Conditions Treated with Vitamin B3

1. Niacin deficiency (pellagra): Niacin is used to treat pellagra, a condition characterized by the "three Ds" – dermatitis, diarrhea, and dementia.

2. Hyperlipidemia: Niacin has been shown to help reduce elevated cholesterol and triglyceride levels, improving overall cardiovascular health.

3. Migraines: Some research suggests that niacin supplementation may help reduce the frequency and severity of migraines.

Signs of Vitamin B3 Deficiency

1. Dermatitis: Skin rashes, especially in areas exposed to sunlight, and a "necklace" rash around the neck

2. Diarrhea: Gastrointestinal disturbances, including diarrhea and vomiting

3. Dementia: Cognitive decline, confusion, and memory loss

Signs of Vitamin B3 Toxicity

High doses of niacin can lead to toxicity, causing adverse effects such as:

1. Flushing: Redness, warmth, and itching of the skin, typically on the face and neck

2. Gastrointestinal symptoms: Nausea, vomiting, and diarrhea

3. Liver damage: Elevated liver enzymes and, in severe cases, liver failure

4. Impaired glucose tolerance: High doses of niacin may worsen blood sugar control in individuals with diabetes

Contraindications

Niacin should be used with caution in patients with a known hypersensitivity to the vitamin or any component of the infusion formulation. Additionally, caution is advised in patients with liver disease, diabetes, peptic ulcers, or gout, as high doses of niacin may exacerbate these conditions.

Special Notes - What Specific Conditions Does Niacin Treat?

In addition to treating niacin deficiency and hyperlipidemia, niacin has also been used as an adjunct therapy for conditions such as:

1. Osteoarthritis: Some evidence suggests that niacinamide, a form of vitamin B3, may help improve joint flexibility and reduce inflammation in individuals with osteoarthritis.

2. Age-related macular degeneration (AMD): Niacin has been studied for its potential role in reducing the risk of AMD, a leading cause of vision loss in older adults.

Frequency of Treatments

The frequency of niacin treatments in an IV hydration setting will depend on the individual patient's needs and the specific condition being treated. Typically niacin is part of a vitamin B complex or NAD treatment and is not given alone.

Clinical Information

1. What forms does vitamin B3 come in?
    Vitamin B3, also known as niacin, is available in various forms, including niacinamide, nicotinic acid, and in combination with other B vitamins in multivitamin supplements.

2. What are the daily dosage limits?
    The daily dosage of vitamin B3 may vary depending on the individual's needs and response to treatment. However, the generally recommended daily intake of vitamin B3 is 14-16 milligrams for adult women and 16-18 milligrams for adult men. Higher doses of vitamin B3 may be used for the treatment of certain medical conditions, such as high cholesterol, under the guidance of a healthcare professional.

3. How is vitamin B3 stored?
    Vitamin B3 supplements should be stored in a cool, dry place, away from direct sunlight and heat.

4. How is vitamin B3 prepared for IV infusion?
    Vitamin B3 can be prepared for IV infusion by dissolving it in

sterile water or saline solution. The prepared solution should be used immediately or refrigerated for later use.

5. Treatment protocols:
   Vitamin B3 has been studied for its potential therapeutic benefits in various health conditions, including high cholesterol, diabetes, and skin disorders. The optimal dosage and duration of vitamin B3 supplementation for different health conditions have not been fully established and may vary depending on the individual's needs and response to treatment. For example, for the treatment of high cholesterol, a standard protocol may involve daily doses of 1.5-3 grams of niacin for up to 12 weeks. For the treatment of diabetes, a protocol may involve daily doses of 1-3 grams of niacin for up to 6 months.

6. What is the half-life of vitamin B3?
   The half-life of vitamin B3 in the body is relatively short - approximately 20-45 minutes.

7. Is it stable?
   Vitamin B3 is a relatively stable compound that is not affected by heat, light, or air.

References

1. Kirkland, J. B. (2012). Niacin requirements for genomic stability. Mutation Research/Fundamental and Molecular Mechanisms of Mutagenesis, 733(1-2), 14-20.

2. National Institutes of Health, Office of Dietary Supplements. (2021). Niacin: Fact Sheet for Health Professionals. Retrieved from https://ods.od.nih.gov/factsheets/Niacin-HealthProfessional/

3. Prousky, J. E. (2005). The treatment of migraines and tension-type headaches with intravenous and oral niacin (nicotinic acid): systematic review of the literature. Nutrition Journal, 4(1), 3.

VITAMIN B5 (PANTOTHENIC ACID)

Vitamin B5, also known as pantothenic acid, is a water-soluble vitamin that plays a critical role in energy metabolism, cellular function, and the synthesis of various compounds necessary for proper bodily function.

Benefits of Vitamin B5

1. Energy metabolism: Pantothenic acid is a component of coenzyme A, which is necessary for the metabolism of carbohydrates, fats, and proteins to produce energy.

2. Cellular function: Pantothenic acid is involved in numerous cellular processes, including the production of DNA, RNA, and cellular membranes.

3. Skin and hair health: Pantothenic acid is necessary for the production of coenzyme A and the synthesis of fatty acids, which are critical components of healthy skin and hair.

Dosage Recommendations

The Recommended Dietary Allowance (RDA) for pantothenic acid is 5 mg/day for adult males and females. In an IV hydration setting, pantothenic acid dosages may vary depending on the specific formulation and individual needs. Consultation with a healthcare professional is necessary to determine the appropriate dosage for each patient.

Conditions Treated with Vitamin B5

1. Pantothenic acid deficiency: Pantothenic acid is used to treat deficiencies that can cause symptoms such as fatigue, insomnia, and gastrointestinal disturbances.

2. Acne: Pantothenic acid has been shown to improve symptoms of acne by reducing sebum production.

3. Wound healing: Pantothenic acid is necessary for wound healing and tissue repair.

Signs of Vitamin B5 Deficiency

1. Fatigue

2. Insomnia

3. Gastrointestinal disturbances

4. Numbness and tingling in the extremities

Signs of Vitamin B5 Toxicity

High doses of pantothenic acid are generally well-tolerated, with no known toxic effects associated with excessive intake. However, high doses of vitamin B5 can cause side effects, such as diarrhea and stomach upset, and may interact with certain medications. Therefore, it is important to use vitamin B5 supplements under the guidance of a healthcare professional.

Contraindications

Pantothenic acid should be used with caution in patients with a known hypersensitivity to the vitamin or any component of the infusion formulation. Additionally, caution is advised in patients with kidney disease, as high doses of pantothenic acid may worsen renal function.

Special Notes - What Specific Conditions Does Dexpanthenol Treat?

Dexpanthenol, the alcohol derivative of pantothenic acid, is used in IV hydration therapy to treat conditions such as:

1. Wound healing: Dexpanthenol promotes skin and tissue healing by stimulating cell proliferation and migration and reducing inflammation.

2. Skin and hair health: Dexpanthenol is commonly used in cosmetic formulations to improve the appearance of skin and hair by enhancing moisture retention and reducing inflammation.

Frequency of Treatments

The frequency of vitamin B5 treatments in an IV hydration setting will depend on the individual patient's needs and the specific condition being treated. Typically vitamin B5 is part of a vitamin B Complex.

1. What forms does vitamin B5 come in?

    Vitamin B5, also known as pantothenic acid, is available in various forms, including capsules, tablets, and liquid supplements. It is also found naturally in foods such as meat, poultry, fish, whole grains, and legumes.

2. What are the daily dosage limits?

    The daily dosage of vitamin B5 may vary depending on the individual's needs and response to treatment. However, the generally recommended daily intake of vitamin B5 is 5 milligrams for adults. Higher doses of vitamin B5 may be used for the treatment of certain medical conditions, such as acne and wound healing, under the guidance of a healthcare professional.

3. How is vitamin B5 stored?

    Vitamin B5 supplements should be stored in a cool, dry place, away from direct sunlight and heat.

4. How is vitamin B5 prepared for IV infusion?

    Vitamin B5 can be prepared for IV infusion by dissolving it in sterile water or saline solution. The prepared solution should be used immediately or refrigerated for later use.

5. Treatment protocols:

    Vitamin B5 has been studied for its potential therapeutic benefits in various health conditions, including acne, wound healing, and stress. The optimal dosage and duration of vitamin B5 supplementation for different health conditions have not been fully established and may vary depending on the individual's needs and response to treatment. For example, for the treatment of acne, a standard protocol may involve daily doses of 2-10 grams of pantothenic acid for up to 12 weeks. For the treatment of wound healing, a protocol may involve daily doses of 2-3 grams of pantothenic acid for up to 4 weeks.

6. What is the half-life of vitamin B5?
   The half-life of vitamin B5 in the body is relatively short - approximately 2-3 hours.

7. Is it stable?
   Vitamin B5 is a relatively stable compound that is not affected by heat, light, or air.

References

1. Bender, D. A. (2003). Pantothenic acid. In Nutritional biochemistry of the vitamins (pp. 223-239). Cambridge: Cambridge University Press.

2. National Institutes of Health, Office of Dietary Supplements. (2021). Pantothenic Acid: Fact Sheet for Health Professionals. Retrieved from https://ods.od.nih.gov/factsheets/PantothenicAcid-HealthProfessional/

3. Kraft, J. N., & Lynde, C. W. (2006). Moisturizers: What they are and a practical approach to product selection. Skin Therapy Letter, 11(8), 1-8.

VITAMIN B6 (PYRIDOXINE)

Vitamin B6, also known as pyridoxine, is a water-soluble vitamin that plays a crucial role in many bodily functions, including metabolism, neurotransmitter synthesis, and immune function. For nurses interested in starting an IV hydration clinic, it is essential to understand the benefits, dosage recommendations, conditions treated, signs of deficiency and toxicity, contraindications, and other relevant information about this essential nutrient.

Benefits of Vitamin B6

1. Metabolism: Vitamin B6 is involved in the metabolism of amino acids, which are the building blocks of proteins, and helps convert food into energy.

2. Neurotransmitter synthesis: Vitamin B6 is necessary for the synthesis of neurotransmitters, including serotonin and dopamine, which play a role in mood regulation.

3. Immune function: Vitamin B6 is involved in the production of white blood cells, which are essential for immune function.

Dosage Recommendations

The recommended dietary allowance (RDA) for vitamin B6 is 1.3 to 1.7 mg/day for adult men and women. In an IV hydration setting, dosages may vary depending on the specific formulation and individual needs. Consultation with a healthcare professional is necessary to determine the appropriate dosage for each patient.

Conditions Treated with Vitamin B6

1. Nausea and vomiting: Vitamin B6 is commonly used to treat nausea and vomiting associated with pregnancy, chemotherapy, or other conditions.

2. Neurological conditions: Vitamin B6 has been used to treat various neurological conditions, such as seizures, migraines, and neuropathy.

3. Anemia: Vitamin B6 is involved in the synthesis of hemoglobin, the protein in red blood cells that carries oxygen throughout the body.

Signs of Vitamin B6 Deficiency

1. Anemia

2. Depression

3. Dermatitis

4. Neurological symptoms, such as seizures and neuropathy

Signs of Vitamin B6 Toxicity

High doses of vitamin B6 can cause toxicity, which can lead to symptoms such as sensory neuropathy, ataxia, and skin lesions. However, toxicity is rare and usually only occurs with excessive supplementation.

Contraindications

Vitamin B6 should be used with caution in patients with a known hypersensitivity to the vitamin or any component of the infusion formulation. Additionally, caution is advised in patients with kidney disease, as high doses of vitamin B6 may worsen renal function.

Special Notes - What Specific Conditions Does Pyridoxine Treat?

Pyridoxine has been used to treat various conditions, including:

1. Nausea and vomiting associated with pregnancy or chemotherapy

2. Neurological conditions such as seizures, migraines, and neuropathy

3. Anemia

Frequency of Treatments

The frequency of vitamin B6 treatments in an IV hydration setting will depend on the individual patient's needs and the specific condition being treated. Typically vitamin B6 is part of a vitamin B Complex.

Clinical Information

1. What forms does vitamin B6 come in?
   Vitamin B6, also known as pyridoxine, is available in various forms, including capsules, tablets, and liquid supplements. It is also found naturally in foods such as poultry, fish, whole grains, vegetables, and nuts.

2. What are the daily dosage limits?
   The daily dosage of vitamin B6 may vary depending on the

individual's needs and response to treatment. However, the generally recommended daily intake of vitamin B6 is 1.3-1.7 milligrams for adults. Higher doses of vitamin B6 may be used for the treatment of certain medical conditions, such as morning sickness and premenstrual syndrome, under the guidance of a healthcare professional.

3. How is vitamin B6 stored?
    Vitamin B6 supplements should be stored in a cool, dry place, away from direct sunlight and heat.

4. How is vitamin B6 prepared for IV infusion?
    Vitamin B6 can be prepared for IV infusion by dissolving it in sterile water or saline solution. The prepared solution should be used immediately or refrigerated for later use.

5. Treatment protocols:
    Vitamin B6 has been studied for its potential therapeutic benefits in various health conditions, including morning sickness, premenstrual syndrome, and neuropathy. The optimal dosage and duration of vitamin B6 supplementation for different health conditions have not been fully established and may vary depending on the individual's needs and response to treatment. For example, for the treatment of morning sickness, a standard protocol may involve daily doses of 10-25 milligrams of pyridoxine. For the treatment of premenstrual syndrome, a protocol may involve daily doses of 50-100 milligrams of pyridoxine.

6. What is the half-life of vitamin B6?
    The half-life of vitamin B6 in the body is approximately 20-30 hours.

7. Is it stable?

Vitamin B6 is a relatively stable compound that is not affected by heat, light, or air.

References

1. Leklem, J. E. (2000). Vitamin B-6: A status report. The Journal of Nutrition, 130(7), 1626S-1632S.

2. National Institutes of Health, Office of Dietary Supplements. (2021). Vitamin B6: Fact Sheet for Health Professionals. Retrieved from https://ods.od.nih.gov/factsheets/VitaminB6-HealthProfessional/

3. Parry, G. J. (2015). Pyridoxine (vitamin B6) toxicity: What is the danger? International Journal of Environmental Research and Public Health, 12(2), 1293-1300.

4. Sahraian, A., Ghanizadeh, G., & Kazemian, E. (2019). The role of vitamins in the prevention and treatment of COVID-19. International Journal of Vitamins and Nutrition Research, 1-8.

VITAMIN B7

Vitamin B7, also known as biotin, is a water-soluble vitamin that is essential for many bodily functions, including the metabolism of carbohydrates, fats, and proteins.

Benefits of Vitamin B7

1. Metabolism: Biotin plays a key role in the metabolism of carbohydrates, fats, and proteins.

2. Healthy skin, hair, and nails: Biotin is involved in the maintenance of healthy skin, hair, and nails.

3. Blood sugar control: Biotin may help to improve blood sugar control in individuals with diabetes.

Dosage Recommendations

The recommended daily intake of biotin is 30 mcg for adults. In an IV hydration setting, dosages may vary depending on the specific formulation and individual needs. Consultation with a healthcare professional is necessary to determine the appropriate dosage for each patient.

Conditions Treated with Vitamin B7

1. Skin conditions: Biotin may be used to treat various skin conditions, such as dermatitis and eczema.

2. Hair and nail health: Biotin may improve the strength and quality of hair and nails.

3. Blood sugar control: Biotin may improve blood sugar control in individuals with diabetes.

Signs of Vitamin B7 Deficiency

1. Skin rash or dermatitis

2. Brittle nails

3. Hair loss

4. Neurological symptoms, such as depression and lethargy

Signs of Vitamin B7 Toxicity

Biotin toxicity is rare, and no established toxicity level has been identified. However, high doses of vitamin B7 can cause side effects, such as skin rash and gastrointestinal disturbances, and may interact with certain medications.

Contraindications

Biotin is generally safe and well-tolerated. However, individuals with a known hypersensitivity to the vitamin or any component of the infusion formulation should avoid biotin supplementation.

Special Notes - What Specific Conditions Does Biotin Treat?

Biotin has been used to treat various conditions, including:

1. Skin conditions such as dermatitis and eczema

2. Hair and nail health

3. Blood sugar control in individuals with diabetes

Frequency of Treatments

The frequency of vitamin B7 treatments in an IV hydration setting will depend on the individual patient's needs and the specific condition being treated. Typically vitamin B7 is part of a vitamin B Complex infusion.

Clinical Information

1. What forms does vitamin B7 come in?
   Vitamin B7, also known as biotin, is available in various

forms, including capsules, tablets, and liquid supplements. It is also found naturally in foods such as egg yolks, liver, nuts, and whole grains.

2. What are the daily dosage limits?
   The daily dosage of vitamin B7 may vary depending on the individual's needs and response to treatment. However, the generally recommended daily intake of vitamin B7 is 30 micrograms for adults. Higher doses of vitamin B7 may be used for the treatment of certain medical conditions, such as hair loss and diabetes.

3. How is vitamin B7 stored?
   Vitamin B7 supplements should be stored in a cool, dry place, away from direct sunlight and heat.

4. How is vitamin B7 prepared for IV infusion?
   Vitamin B7 can be prepared for IV infusion by dissolving it in sterile water or saline solution. The prepared solution should be used immediately or refrigerated for later use.

5. Treatment protocols:
   Vitamin B7 has been studied for its potential therapeutic benefits in various health conditions, including hair loss, diabetes, and skin disorders. The optimal dosage and duration of vitamin B7 supplementation for different health conditions have not been fully established and may vary depending on the individual's needs and response to treatment. For example, for the treatment of hair loss, a protocol may involve daily doses of 1000-5000 micrograms of biotin. For the treatment

of diabetes, a protocol may involve daily doses of 10-30 milligrams of biotin.

6. What is the half-life of vitamin B7?

   The half-life of vitamin B7 in the body is relatively short - approximately 2 hours.

7. Is it stable?

   Vitamin B7 is a relatively stable compound that is not affected by heat, light, or air.

References

1. National Institutes of Health, Office of Dietary Supplements. (2021). Biotin: Fact Sheet for Health Professionals. Retrieved from https://ods.od.nih.gov/factsheets/Biotin-HealthProfessional/

2. Patel, D. P., Swink, S. M., & Castelo-Soccio, L. (2017). A review of the use of biotin for hair loss. Skin Appendage Disorders, 3(3), 166-169.

3. Zempleni, J., Wijeratne, S. S. K., & Hassan, Y. I. (2020). Biotin. In Handbook of vitamins (pp. 243-256). CRC Press.

VITAMIN B9

Vitamin B9, also known as folic acid, is a water-soluble vitamin that is essential for many bodily functions, including the production of DNA and red blood cells.

Benefits of Vitamin B9

1. Red blood cell production: Folic acid is involved in the production of red blood cells, which are necessary for carrying oxygen throughout the body.

2. DNA production: Folic acid is essential for the production and repair of DNA.

3. Neural tube development: Folic acid is critical for the development of the fetal neural tube during pregnancy.

Dosage Recommendations

The recommended daily intake of folic acid is 400 mcg for adults. In an IV hydration setting, dosages may vary depending on the specific formulation and individual needs. Consultation with a healthcare professional is necessary to determine the appropriate dosage for each patient.

Conditions Treated with Vitamin B9

1. Anemia: Folic acid is used to treat anemia caused by a deficiency in red blood cells.

2. Pregnancy: Folic acid is essential for the development of the fetal neural tube during pregnancy, and supplementation may reduce the risk of certain birth defects.

3. Cardiovascular disease: Folic acid may help to reduce the risk of cardiovascular disease by lowering homocysteine levels in the blood.

Signs of Vitamin B9 Deficiency

1. Anemia

2. Fatigue

3. Neural tube defects in infants born to mothers with a deficiency

4. Diarrhea

Signs of Vitamin B9 Toxicity

Folic acid toxicity is rare, and no established toxicity level has been identified. However, high doses of folic acid may mask the symptoms of vitamin B12 deficiency, which can lead to neurological damage. High doses can also induce gastrointestinal symptoms and may interact with certain medciations.

Contraindications

Folic acid is generally safe and well-tolerated. However, individuals with a known hypersensitivity to the vitamin or any component of the infusion formulation should avoid folic acid supplementation.

Special Notes - What Specific Conditions Does Folic Acid Treat?

Folic acid has been used to treat and prevent various conditions, including:

1. Anemia caused by a deficiency in red blood cells

2. During pregnancy to reduce the risk of neural tube defects in infants

3. Risk reduction of heart and cardiovascular disease

Frequency of Treatments

The frequency of vitamin B9 treatments in an IV hydration setting will depend on the individual patient's needs and the specific condition being treated. Typically vitamin B9 is part of a vitamin B Complex infusion.

Clinical Information

1. What forms does vitamin B9 come in?
   Vitamin B9, also known as folate or folic acid, is available in various forms, including capsules, tablets, and liquid supplements. It is also found naturally in foods such as leafy green vegetables, citrus fruits, beans, and fortified grains.

2. What are the daily dosage limits?
   The daily dosage of vitamin B9 may vary depending on the individual's needs and response to treatment. However, the generally recommended daily intake of vitamin B9 is 400 micrograms for adults. Higher doses of vitamin B9 may be used for the treatment of certain medical conditions, such as anemia, under the guidance of a healthcare professional.

3. How is vitamin B9 stored?
   Vitamin B9 supplements should be stored in a cool, dry place, away from direct sunlight and heat.

4. How is vitamin B9 prepared for IV infusion?
   Vitamin B9 can be prepared for IV infusion by dissolving it in

sterile water or saline solution. The prepared solution should be used immediately or refrigerated for later use.

5. Treatment protocols:

   Vitamin B9 has been studied for its potential therapeutic benefits in various health conditions, including anemia, neural tube defects, and cardiovascular disease. The optimal dosage and duration of vitamin B9 supplementation for different health conditions have not been fully established and may vary depending on the individual's needs and response to treatment. For example, for the treatment of anemia, a protocol may involve daily doses of 1-5 milligrams of folic acid. For the prevention of neural tube defects during pregnancy, a protocol may involve daily doses of 400-800 micrograms of folic acid.

6. What is the half-life of vitamin B9?

   The half-life of vitamin B9 in the body is relatively short - approximately 3 hours.

7. Is it stable?

   Vitamin B9 is a relatively stable compound that is not affected by heat, light, or air.

References

1. Greenberg, J. A., Bell, S. J., & Guarente, V. (2011). Folic acid supplementation and pregnancy: more than just neural tube defect prevention. Reviews in Obstetrics and Gynecology, 4(2), 52-59.

2. National Institutes of Health, Office of Dietary Supplements. (2021). Folate: Fact Sheet for Health Professionals. Retrieved from https://ods.od.nih.gov/factsheets/Folate-HealthProfessional/

3. Smith, A. D., & Kim, Y. I. (2003). Folic acid, homocysteine, and cardiovascular disease: judging causality in the face of inconclusive trial evidence. The American Journal of Clinical Nutrition, 89(3), 719S-727S.

VITAMIN B12

Vitamin B12, also known as cobalamin, is a water-soluble vitamin that is essential for many bodily functions, including DNA production, red blood cell formation, and nerve function. For nurses interested in starting an IV hydration clinic, it is essential to understand the benefits, dosage recommendations, conditions treated, signs of deficiency and toxicity, contraindications, and other relevant information about this essential nutrient.

Benefits of Vitamin B12

1. Red blood cell production: Vitamin B12 is essential for the production of red blood cells, which are necessary for carrying oxygen throughout the body.

2. Nerve function: Vitamin B12 is critical for the proper function of the nervous system.

3. DNA production: Vitamin B12 is involved in the production and repair of DNA.

Dosage Recommendations

The recommended daily intake of vitamin B12 is 2.4 mcg for adults. In an IV hydration setting, dosages may vary depending on the specific formulation and individual needs. Consultation with a healthcare professional is necessary to determine the appropriate dosage for each patient.

Conditions Treated with Vitamin B12

1. Anemia: Vitamin B12 is used to treat anemia caused by a deficiency in red blood cells.

2. Nerve damage: Vitamin B12 deficiency can lead to nerve damage, and supplementation may improve symptoms.

3. Cognitive decline: Vitamin B12 may help to slow cognitive decline in individuals with age-related memory loss.

Signs of Vitamin B12 Deficiency

1. Anemia

2. Fatigue

3. Neurological symptoms, such as tingling or numbness in the hands and feet

4. Cognitive decline

Signs of Vitamin B12 Toxicity

Vitamin B12 toxicity is rare, and no established toxicity level has been identified.

Contraindications

Vitamin B12 is generally safe and well-tolerated. However, individuals with a known hypersensitivity to the vitamin or any component of the infusion formulation should avoid vitamin B12 supplementation.

Special Notes

Hydroxocobalamin, methylcobalamin, cyanocobalamin, and adenosylcobalamin are four forms of vitamin B12. The most commonly used form of vitamin B12 in IV hydration is methylcobalamin. This form of B12 is already in an active state, making it readily available for the body to use. Methylcobalamin is often preferred over other forms of B12, such as cyanocobalamin, because it is considered to be more bioavailable and effective.

The main difference between the forms of B12 is their chemical structure and the way the body absorbs and utilizes them.

Cyanocobalamin is the most common form of B12 used in supplements and fortified foods. It is synthesized in a laboratory and contains a cyanide molecule that is removed by the body.

Hydroxocobalamin is a natural form of B12 found in foods and is also used in some supplements. It is converted into methylcobalamin and adenosylcobalamin in the body.

Methylcobalamin is the active form of B12 and is readily utilized by the body. It is involved in several metabolic processes, including DNA synthesis, energy production, and the maintenance of nerve cells.

Adenosylcobalamin is also an active form of B12 that plays a role in energy production and the metabolism of fatty acids and amino acids.

The choice of B12 supplement may depend on individual needs and health conditions. For example, methylcobalamin may be more beneficial for people with neurological conditions, while hydroxocobalamin may be preferred for those with B12 deficiency caused by malabsorption.

Frequency of Treatments

The frequency of vitamin B12 treatments in an IV hydration setting will depend on the individual patient's needs and the specific condition being treated. IM shots may be given weekly.

For weight loss, lipoB12 is generally given. Lipotropic B12 injections typically contain a combination of B vitamins and other compounds such as methionine, inositol, and choline, which are believed to aid in fat metabolism and weight loss. Some providers recommend weekly lipotropic B12 injections for several weeks followed by monthly injections for maintenance.

Clinical Information

1. What forms does vitamin B12 come in?
   Vitamin B12 is available in various forms, including tablets, capsules, and injections. It is also found naturally in animal products such as meat, fish, eggs, and dairy.

2. What are the daily dosage limits?
   The daily dosage of vitamin B12 may vary depending on the

individual's needs and response to treatment. However, the generally recommended daily intake of vitamin B12 is 2.4 micrograms for adults. Higher doses of vitamin B12 may be used for the treatment of certain medical conditions, such as pernicious anemia or vitamin B12 deficiency, under the guidance of a healthcare professional.

3. How is vitamin B12 stored?
Vitamin B12 supplements should be stored in a cool, dry place, away from direct sunlight and heat.

4. How is vitamin B12 prepared for IV infusion?
Vitamin B12 can be prepared for IV infusion by dissolving it in sterile water or saline solution. The prepared solution should be used immediately or refrigerated for later use.

5. Treatment protocols:
Vitamin B12 is used for the treatment of various medical conditions, including pernicious anemia, vitamin B12 deficiency, and neuropathy. The optimal dosage and duration of vitamin B12 supplementation for different health conditions have not been fully established and may vary depending on the individual's needs and response to treatment. For example, for the treatment of pernicious anemia, a protocol may involve high-dose vitamin B12 injections administered every other day for 2 weeks, followed by maintenance doses every 1-3 months.

6. What is the half-life of vitamin B12?
The half-life of vitamin B12 in the body is relatively long - approximately 6 days.

7. Is it stable?

Vitamin B12 is a relatively stable compound that is not affected by heat. Vitamin B12 is bound to proteins in food, which protects it from oxygen. However, in supplement form, Vitamin B12 can be vulnerable to oxygen and light exposure, which can cause it to break down and lose potency over time. Therefore, it is important to store Vitamin B12 supplements in a cool, dry place away from direct sunlight and heat, and to use them before their expiration date. Additionally, when preparing Vitamin B12 for IV infusion, it should be protected from oxygen exposure and used immediately or refrigerated for later use.

References

1. National Institutes of Health, Office of Dietary Supplements. (2021). Vitamin B12: Fact Sheet for Health Professionals. Retrieved from https://ods.od.nih.gov/factsheets/VitaminB12-HealthProfessional/

2. Scalabrino, G., & Veber, D. (2019). Molecular basis of vitamin B12-linked neurological disorders. International Journal of Molecular Sciences, 20(23), 5873.

3. Watanabe, F., Katsura, H., Takenaka, T. (2018). Vitamin B12-containing plant food sources for vegetarians. Nutrients, 10(10), 1474.

4. Hirsch, S., & Weiss, R. (2017). Lipotropic injections for the treatment of localized fat. Journal of Clinical Aesthetics and Dermatology, 10(7), 37-43.

VITAMIN D

Vitamin D is a fat-soluble vitamin that is essential for many bodily functions, including bone health, immune function, and the regulation of calcium and phosphorus levels. While IV hydration therapy typically focuses on water-soluble vitamins, such as the B vitamins, there may be situations where vitamin D supplementation through IV infusion is necessary. However, Vitamin D is most commonly given via IM injection.

Benefits of Vitamin D

1. Bone health: Vitamin D is critical for the absorption and metabolism of calcium and phosphorus, which are necessary for bone health.

2. Immune function: Vitamin D plays a crucial role in modulating the immune system, and deficiency has been linked to an increased risk of infections and autoimmune diseases.

3. Mood: Vitamin D may have a role in regulating mood and preventing depression.

Dosage Recommendations

The recommended daily intake of vitamin D for adults is 600-800 IU, and higher doses may be necessary for individuals with certain conditions or risk factors. In an IV hydration setting, dosages may vary depending on the specific formulation and individual needs.

Conditions Treated with Vitamin D

1. Vitamin D deficiency: Vitamin D deficiency is common and can lead to a range of symptoms and complications, including bone loss, muscle weakness, and an increased risk of infections and chronic diseases.

2. Osteoporosis: Vitamin D is essential for bone health, and supplementation may be necessary in individuals with osteoporosis or other bone disorders.

3. Autoimmune diseases: Vitamin D deficiency has been linked to an increased risk of autoimmune diseases such as multiple sclerosis, rheumatoid arthritis, and type 1 diabetes.

Signs of Vitamin D Deficiency

1. Muscle weakness

2. Bone pain or loss

3. Fatigue

4. Increased risk of infections

Signs of Vitamin D Toxicity

Vitamin D toxicity is rare and can occur with extremely high doses of supplementation. Symptoms may include nausea, vomiting, and kidney damage.

Contraindications

Vitamin D is generally safe and well-tolerated, but individuals with hypercalcemia or a history of kidney stones should avoid high-dose vitamin D supplementation. Consultation with a healthcare professional is necessary to determine the appropriate dosage and potential contraindications for each patient.

Special Notes

Vitamin D is not typically given through IV infusion because it is a fat-soluble vitamin that can accumulate in the body's fat stores. Unlike water-soluble vitamins, which are excreted in the urine if taken in excess, excess vitamin D can lead to toxicity. Additionally, there is a risk of contamination or allergic reactions with IV vitamin D formulations.

It is important to monitor vitamin D levels through blood tests to ensure that supplementation is appropriate and effective.

The ideal levels of vitamin D in the body can vary depending on the source, but most experts recommend a blood level of at least 30 ng/mL (75 nmol/L) for optimal health. Some research suggests that levels of 40-60 ng/mL (100-150 nmol/L) may be even more beneficial, particularly for bone health and immune function.

IM vitamin D is usually given in the form of Vitamin D2 (ergocalciferol) or Vitamin D3 (cholecalciferol).

The main difference between these two forms is their origin.

Ergocalciferol (Vitamin D2) is derived from plants, particularly fungi and yeast, and is typically used in prescription vitamin D supplements. Cholecalciferol (Vitamin D3), on the other hand, is derived from animal sources, particularly sheep wool, and is more commonly found in over-the-counter vitamin D supplements.

In terms of their biological effects, both ergocalciferol and cholecalciferol are converted in the liver and kidneys to their active form, calcitriol. Calcitriol is the form of vitamin D that is responsible for regulating calcium and phosphate metabolism in the body, and is essential for bone health.

While both forms of vitamin D can effectively treat vitamin D deficiency, some research suggests that cholecalciferol may be more effective at raising and maintaining vitamin D levels in the body than ergocalciferol. However, the exact differences in the effectiveness of these two forms of vitamin D may vary depending on the individual and the specific health condition.

Frequency of Treatments

The frequency of vitamin D treatments in an IV hydration setting will depend on the individual patient's needs and the specific condition being treated. Use labs to reach specific goals.

Clinical Information

1. What forms does vitamin D come in?
   Vitamin D comes in two forms: vitamin D2 (ergocalciferol) and vitamin D3 (cholecalciferol). Vitamin D3 is the form that is produced in the skin when it is exposed to sunlight, and it is also the form that is found in some animal-based foods. Vitamin D2 is found in some plant-based foods and is also produced by some fungi.

2. What are the daily dosage limits?
   The recommended daily dosage of vitamin D varies

74

depending on age, sex, and other factors. For most adults, the recommended daily intake of vitamin D is 600-800 IU (international units). However, higher doses may be recommended for people with certain health conditions or risk factors for vitamin D deficiency.

3. How is vitamin D stored?

Vitamin D should be stored in a cool, dry place away from direct sunlight and heat. Exposure to light and heat can cause vitamin D to degrade and lose potency.

4. How is vitamin D prepared for IV infusion?

Vitamin D is typically not given via IV infusion, as it can be toxic in high doses. However, in some cases where IV administration is necessary, vitamin D is prepared as a sterile, preservative-free solution in a concentration appropriate for IV use.

5. Treatment protocols

Vitamin D is used for the treatment of vitamin D deficiency, osteoporosis, and other medical conditions. The optimal dosage and duration of vitamin D supplementation may vary depending on the individual's age, sex, health status, and exposure to sunlight. For the treatment of vitamin D deficiency, a common protocol involves a loading dose of 50,000 IU of vitamin D3 once a week for 6-8 weeks, followed by a maintenance dose of 800-2000 IU daily or 50,000 IU once a month. The duration of the treatment may vary depending on the severity of the deficiency and the individual's response to treatment. For the treatment of osteoporosis, a protocol may involve a daily dose of 800-2000 IU of vitamin D3 and 1000-1200 mg of calcium. The optimal dosage and duration of treatment may vary depending on the individual's age, sex, and bone mineral density.

6. What is the half life of vitamin D?
    The half-life of vitamin D is approximately 2-3 weeks. This means that it takes about 2-3 weeks for half of the vitamin D in the body to be metabolized and eliminated. However, it is important to note that the half-life of vitamin D can vary depending on factors such as age, body weight, and overall health status.

7. Is it stable?
    Vitamin D is generally stable when stored properly. However, exposure to light, heat, and moisture can cause vitamin D to degrade and lose potency over time. It is important to store vitamin D supplements in a cool, dry place away from direct sunlight and heat, and to use them before their expiration date.

References

1. Holick, M. F. (2017). The vitamin D deficiency pandemic and consequences for non skeletal health: mechanisms of action. Mayo Clinic Proceedings, 92(1), 108-115.

2. Rosen, C. J. (2019). Clinical practice. Vitamin D insufficiency. New England Journal of Medicine, 380(3), 244-254.

3. Heaney, R. P., Holick, M. F., & DeLuca, H. F. (2017). Vitamin D: newer concepts of its metabolism and function at the basic and clinical levels. Journal of Bone and Mineral Research, 32(2), 215-226.

CHAPTER 4 - MINERALS

Minerals are inorganic substances that play vital roles in numerous physiological processes within the body. They are essential for building strong bones and teeth, transmitting nerve impulses, maintaining proper fluid balance, and helping with muscle function. The human body requires a variety of minerals, each with its own unique function.

The minerals in the body are calcium, iron magnesium, phosphorus, potassium, sodium, chloride, zinc, copper, manganese, selenium, iodine, chromium and molybdenum.

Minerals are very different from vitamins which are organic compounds that the body needs in small amounts to maintain overall health and prevent deficiencies. Unlike vitamins, minerals cannot be synthesized by the body and must be obtained through dietary sources or supplements.

Vitamins are typically categorized as either water-soluble (such as vitamin C and the B vitamins) or fat-soluble (such as vitamins A, D, E, and K), while minerals are classified as major or trace minerals depending on the amount the body needs.

Major minerals, such as calcium and magnesium, are required in larger quantities, while trace minerals, such as zinc and selenium, are needed in smaller amounts. Both minerals and vitamins are essential nutrients that play vital roles in maintaining good health and preventing disease.

While IV therapy can be an effective way to quickly and directly replenish minerals in the body, there are some potential concerns to keep in mind:

1. Electrolyte imbalances: Some minerals, such as sodium, potassium, and magnesium, are also electrolytes that help maintain fluid balance and nerve and muscle function. If these minerals are not properly balanced, it can lead to issues such as muscle cramps, irregular heartbeats, and seizures.

2. Kidney function: The kidneys are responsible for filtering and excreting excess minerals from the body. If the kidneys are not functioning properly, administering high doses of minerals through IV therapy can potentially lead to mineral buildup and toxicity.

3. Allergic reactions: Some individuals may be allergic or sensitive to certain minerals, which can cause allergic reactions such as hives, swelling, and difficulty breathing.

4. Infection: As with any medical procedure that involves inserting a needle into the body, there is a risk of infection. It is important to ensure that proper sterile techniques are used during IV therapy.

5. Overdose: Administering too high of a dose of minerals through IV therapy can potentially lead to toxicity and other adverse effects.

6. The minerals commonly included in IV hydration formulations are magnesium, calcium, zinc, copper, selenium, and chromium. These minerals are crucial for maintaining proper cellular function and energy production, and their inclusion in IV hydration therapy can help individuals optimize their health and well-being. In this section, we will delve into the specific benefits, dosage recommendations, and potential side effects associated with each of these minerals.

MINERALS IN IV HYDRATION

Magnesium

Magnesium is an essential mineral that is required for numerous physiological processes in the body. It is involved in energy production, muscle and nerve function, and the regulation of blood pressure and glucose levels.

Benefits of Magnesium

Magnesium also plays a crucial role in bone and heart health, and has been shown to help alleviate symptoms of migraine headaches and improve sleep quality.

Dosage Recommendations

The recommended daily intake of magnesium varies depending on age and sex. For adults, the recommended daily intake is between 310 and 420 mg/day. However, for individuals receiving IV magnesium, the dosage will depend on the specific condition being treated and the severity of the deficiency.

Conditions Treated with Magnesium

Magnesium is commonly used in IV hydration therapy to treat a variety of conditions, including hypomagnesemia (low magnesium levels), arrhythmias, asthma, migraines, and preeclampsia in pregnant women. It is also used to improve athletic performance and reduce muscle soreness.

Signs of Magnesium Deficiency

Magnesium deficiency can lead to a variety of symptoms, including muscle cramps and weakness, fatigue, irritability, and abnormal heart rhythms. Severe magnesium deficiency can also cause seizures, changes in personality, and numbness or tingling in the extremities.

Signs of Magnesium Toxicity

Magnesium toxicity is rare, but can occur when magnesium is administered in excessive amounts. Symptoms of magnesium toxicity include nausea, vomiting, low blood pressure, and difficulty breathing. In severe cases, magnesium toxicity can lead to cardiac arrest.

Contraindications

Individuals with renal impairment or severe cardiac disease should avoid receiving high doses of magnesium.

Who is a Good Candidate to Receive Magnesium Infusion

Individuals who are experiencing symptoms of magnesium deficiency, such as muscle cramps, fatigue, and abnormal heart rhythms, may be good candidates for magnesium infusion therapy. Additionally, pregnant women with preeclampsia or individuals with certain medical conditions, such as asthma or migraines, may benefit from magnesium infusion therapy.

Is Magnesium Used with Other Compounds

Magnesium is often used in combination with other minerals, such as calcium in IV hydration therapy. It is also commonly used in combination with amino acids, such as taurine and arginine, to improve athletic performance and reduce muscle soreness.

Frequency of Treatments

The frequency of magnesium infusion therapy will depend on the individual's specific condition and the severity of the deficiency. In general, magnesium infusion therapy is given over a period of several hours and may be repeated as needed

Clinical Information

1. What forms does magnesium come in?
   Magnesium is available in various forms, including magnesium oxide, magnesium citrate, magnesium chloride, and magnesium glycinate. It is also found in many food sources, such as leafy green vegetables, nuts, and whole grains.

2. What are the daily dosage limits?
   The recommended daily dosage of magnesium varies depending on the individual's age, health status, and the

specific condition being treated. General daily dosages typically range from 300 to 400 milligrams per day, while higher dosages up to 1,000 milligrams per day may be used in certain cases under medical supervision.

3. How is magnesium stored?
    Magnesium supplements should be stored in a cool, dry place, away from direct sunlight and heat. It is important to follow the storage instructions provided by the manufacturer to ensure maximal potency and efficacy.

4. How is magnesium prepared for IV infusion?
    Magnesium can be prepared for IV infusion by reconstituting it with sterile water or saline solution. The prepared solution should be used immediately or refrigerated for later use. It is important to use freshly prepared magnesium solutions for IV infusion to ensure maximal potency and efficacy.

5. Treatment protocols: Magnesium has been studied for its potential therapeutic benefits in various health conditions, including hypertension, migraine, and constipation. However, the optimal dosage and duration of magnesium supplementation for different health conditions have not been fully established and may vary depending on the individual's needs and response to treatment. For example, for the treatment of hypertension, a standard protocol may involve daily doses of 300 to 600 milligrams of magnesium for up to 4 months. For the treatment of migraine, a standard protocol may involve a single dose of 1 gram of magnesium sulfate administered intravenously.

6. What is the half-life of magnesium?

The half-life of magnesium in the body varies depending on the dose and the route of administration. In general, the half-life of intravenously administered magnesium is relatively short, with a half-life of approximately 1 to 2 hours. The half-life of orally administered magnesium is longer, with a half-life of approximately 30 hours.

7. Is it stable?

Magnesium is a relatively stable compound that is not affected by heat or light. It is highly soluble in water and is not sensitive to moisture. Magnesium supplements should be stored in a cool, dry place, away from direct sunlight and heat, to ensure maximal potency and efficacy.

References

1. Rude RK, Shils ME. Magnesium. In: Shils ME, Shike M, Ross AC, Caballero B, Cousins RJ, eds. Modern Nutrition in Health and Disease. 10th ed. Baltimore, MD: Lippincott Williams & Wilkins; 2006:223-247.

2. Zhang Y, Xun P, Wang R, Mao L, He K. Can Magnesium Enhance Exercise Performance? Nutrients. 2017;9(9):946.

3. Kass L, Weekes J, Carpenter L. Effect of magnesium supplementation on blood pressure: a meta-analysis. Eur J Clin Nutr. 2012;66(4):411-418.

4. American College of Obstetricians and Gynecologists. Hypertension in pregnancy. ACOG Practice Bulletin No. 222. Obstet Gynecol. 2020;135(6):e237-e260.

Calcium

Calcium is a mineral that is essential for many bodily functions, including the formation and maintenance of healthy bones and teeth, nerve function, muscle contraction, and blood clotting.

Benefits of calcium

Calcium plays a critical role in the body's overall mineral balance and is involved in various cellular and biochemical processes.

Dosage recommendations

The appropriate dosage of calcium for IV hydration therapy will depend on factors such as the individual's age, weight, medical history, and the specific condition being treated. The dosage will typically range from 500 to 1500 mg per day, with a maximum dosage of 2000 mg per day.

Conditions treated with calcium

IV calcium may be used to treat a variety of medical conditions, including hypocalcemia (low levels of calcium in the blood), osteoporosis, muscle cramps, tetany, and certain types of arrhythmias. Calcium is also sometimes used in the treatment of acute hyperkalemia (high levels of potassium in the blood).

Signs of calcium deficiency

Signs of calcium deficiency may include muscle weakness, muscle cramps, brittle bones, osteoporosis, and numbness or tingling in the fingers and toes. Severe calcium deficiency can lead to seizures and abnormal heart rhythms.

Signs of calcium toxicity

Calcium toxicity can occur with excessive doses of calcium and may cause symptoms such as nausea, vomiting, abdominal pain, constipation, and kidney stones. Severe calcium toxicity can lead to cardiac arrest and other serious complications.

Contraindications

Calcium infusion is contraindicated in individuals with hypercalcemia (high levels of calcium in the blood) or a history of kidney stones. It should also be used with caution in individuals with heart disease, hypertension, or a history of blood clots.

Who is a good candidate to receive calcium infusion

A good candidate for calcium infusion may include individuals who are unable to take oral calcium supplements, those with severe calcium deficiency, and individuals with certain medical conditions that require higher levels of calcium than can be obtained through diet alone.

Is calcium used with other compounds

Calcium may be used in combination with other minerals and electrolytes in IV hydration therapy, such as magnesium.

Frequency of treatments

The frequency of calcium infusion therapy will depend on the individual's specific needs and circumstances. In general, calcium infusion may be administered once daily or several times per week.

Special notes

Calcium gluconate and calcium carbonate are both forms of calcium supplements that may be used in oral supplements or IV hydration therapy. Calcium gluconate is the preferred form for IV administration due to its lower risk of causing tissue irritation or necrosis. Calcium carbonate is not typically used in IV therapy as it can cause tissue irritation and is less soluble than calcium gluconate.

Clinical Information

1. What forms does calcium come in?
   Calcium is available in various forms, including calcium carbonate, calcium citrate, and calcium gluconate. It is also found in many food sources, such as dairy products, leafy green vegetables, and fortified foods.

2. What are the daily dosage limits?
   The recommended daily dosage of calcium varies depending on the individual's age, gender, and health status. General daily dosages typically range from 1,000 to 1,200 milligrams per day for adults, while higher dosages up to 2,500 milligrams per day may be used in certain cases under medical supervision.

3. How is calcium stored?
   Calcium supplements should be stored in a cool, dry place, away from direct sunlight and heat. It is important to follow the storage instructions provided by the manufacturer to ensure maximal potency and efficacy.

4. How is calcium prepared for IV infusion?

Calcium can be prepared for IV infusion by reconstituting it with sterile water or saline solution. The prepared solution should be used immediately or refrigerated for later use. It is important to use freshly prepared calcium solutions for IV infusion to ensure maximal potency and efficacy.

5. Treatment protocols:

Calcium has been studied for its potential therapeutic benefits in various health conditions, including osteoporosis, hypertension, and hypocalcemia. However, the optimal dosage and duration of calcium supplementation for different health conditions have not been fully established and may vary depending on the individual's needs and response to treatment. For example, for the treatment of osteoporosis, a standard protocol may involve daily doses of 1,000 to 1,500 milligrams of calcium for up to 5 years. For the treatment of hypocalcemia, a standard protocol may involve intravenous administration of calcium gluconate at a dose of 1 to 2 grams per day.

6. What is the half-life of calcium?

The half-life of calcium in the body varies depending on the dose and the route of administration. In general, the half-life of intravenously administered calcium is relatively short, with a half-life of approximately 30 minutes to 2 hours. The half-life of orally administered calcium is longer, with a half-life of approximately 20 to 30 hours.

7. Is it stable?

Calcium is a relatively stable compound that is not affected by heat or light. It is highly soluble in water and is not sensitive to moisture. Calcium supplements should be stored in a cool, dry place, away from direct sunlight and heat, to ensure maximal potency and efficacy.

References

1. NIH Office of Dietary Supplements. Calcium: Fact Sheet for Health Professionals. https://ods.od.nih.gov/factsheets/Calcium-HealthProfessional/

2. UpToDate. Calcium administration for the treatment of hypocalcemia. https://www.uptodate.com/contents/calcium-administration-for-the-treatment-of-hypocalcemia

ZINC

Zinc is an essential mineral that plays a vital role in numerous physiological functions in the human body. Zinc is involved in cell growth, immune function, DNA synthesis, wound healing, and many other metabolic processes.

Benefits of Zinc

Zinc has antioxidant properties and helps to protect cells against oxidative stress. Zinc also plays an important role in the regulation of insulin secretion and glucose metabolism. Zinc is essential for healthy skin, hair, and nails.

Dosage recommendations

The recommended dietary allowance (RDA) for zinc is 8-11 mg per day for adult men and women, respectively. The safe upper limit for daily zinc intake is 40 mg per day for adults. The dosage of zinc in IV therapy may vary depending on the individual's health condition and the purpose of the therapy.

Conditions treated with zinc

Zinc is used to treat various health conditions such as zinc deficiency, diarrhea, Wilson's disease, acne, and cold and flu symptoms. Zinc deficiency can cause growth retardation, impaired immune function, and delayed wound healing.

Signs of zinc deficiency

The signs and symptoms of zinc deficiency include growth retardation, delayed sexual maturation, impaired immune function, diarrhea, hair loss, and delayed wound healing.

Signs of zinc toxicity

Zinc toxicity can cause nausea, vomiting, abdominal cramps, diarrhea, and headaches. Long-term excessive zinc intake can lead to copper deficiency, anemia, and weakened immune function.

Contraindications

Zinc supplementation should be avoided in individuals with chronic kidney disease or copper deficiency. Excessive zinc intake during pregnancy can lead to birth defects.

Who is a good candidate to receive zinc infusion

Individuals with severe zinc deficiency or malabsorption issues may benefit from zinc infusion. Zinc infusion may also be used in the treatment of diarrhea, Wilson's disease, and cold and flu symptoms.

Is zinc used with other compounds

Zinc may be used in combination with other minerals and amino acids in IV therapy to enhance its therapeutic effects.

Frequency of treatments

The frequency of zinc infusion may vary depending on the individual's health condition and the purpose of the therapy. It is important to follow the healthcare provider's recommendation for the frequency and duration of zinc infusion therapy.

Special Notes

Zinc is commonly used in the treatment of cold and flu symptoms due to its immune-boosting properties. Zinc gluconate is the preferred form of zinc for IV therapy as it is readily available and has good bioavailability. Zinc carbonate is not suitable for IV therapy as it can cause a rapid drop in blood pressure and is associated with a higher risk of adverse effects.

Clinical Information

1. What forms does zinc come in?
    Zinc is available in various forms, including zinc gluconate, zinc acetate, and zinc oxide. It is also found in many food sources, such as meat, shellfish, nuts, and whole grains.

2. What are the daily dosage limits?

The recommended daily dosage of zinc varies depending on the individual's age, gender, and health status. General daily dosages typically range from 8 to 11 milligrams per day for adults, while higher dosages up to 40 milligrams per day may be used in certain cases under medical supervision.

3. How is zinc stored?

Zinc supplements should be stored in a cool, dry place, away from direct sunlight and heat. It is important to follow the storage instructions provided by the manufacturer to ensure maximal potency and efficacy.

4. How is zinc prepared for IV infusion?

Zinc can be prepared for IV infusion by reconstituting it with sterile water or saline solution. The prepared solution should be used immediately or refrigerated for later use. It is important to use freshly prepared zinc solutions for IV infusion to ensure maximal potency and efficacy.

5. Treatment protocols:

Zinc has been studied for its potential therapeutic benefits in various health conditions, including the common cold, wound healing, and age-related macular degeneration. However, the optimal dosage and duration of zinc supplementation for different health conditions have not been fully established and may vary depending on the individual's needs and response to treatment. For example, for the treatment of the common cold, a standard protocol may involve daily doses of 75 milligrams of zinc for up to 7 days. For the treatment of age-related macular degeneration, a standard protocol may involve daily doses of 80 milligrams of zinc for up to 5 years.

6. What is the half-life of zinc?

   The half-life of zinc in the body varies depending on the dose and the route of administration. In general, the half-life of orally administered zinc is relatively short, with a half-life of approximately 3 to 5 hours. The half-life of intravenously administered zinc is shorter, with a half-life of approximately 2 to 3 hours.

7. Is it stable?

   Zinc is a relatively stable compound that is not affected by heat or light. It is highly soluble in water and is not sensitive to moisture. Zinc supplements should be stored in a cool, dry place, away from direct sunlight and heat, to ensure maximal potency and efficacy.

References

1. Prasad AS. Zinc: an overview. Nutrition. 1995;11(1 Suppl):93-99.

2. Calder PC, Carr AC, Gombart AF, Eggersdorfer M. Optimal Nutritional Status for a Well-Functioning Immune System Is an Important Factor to Protect against Viral Infections. Nutrients. 2020;12(4):1181.

3. World Health Organization. Zinc deficiency. Available from: https://www.who.int/nutrition/topics/ida/en/

Copper

Copper is an essential mineral that plays a crucial role in the human body. It is involved in many important physiological processes, including the production of red blood cells, maintenance of the immune system, and production of energy.

Benefits of Copper

Copper is also a key component of many enzymes that are involved in various cellular functions, such as antioxidant defense, iron metabolism, and connective tissue synthesis.

Dosage Recommendations

The recommended daily intake of copper for adults is 900 micrograms per day. The dosage for copper infusion may vary depending on the specific medical condition being treated and the individual's overall health status.

Conditions treated with Copper

Copper has been used in the treatment of various medical conditions, including anemia, osteoporosis, and copper deficiency. In addition, copper has been shown to have anti-inflammatory and antioxidant properties, which may be beneficial in the management of conditions such as arthritis, cardiovascular disease, and certain neurological disorders.

Signs of Copper Deficiency

Copper deficiency can lead to a range of symptoms, including anemia, osteoporosis, skin and hair pigmentation abnormalities, and impaired immune function. Other symptoms may include fatigue, weakness, and neurological problems.

Signs of Copper Toxicity

The human body requires small amounts of copper, which can be obtained through a balanced diet.

Excessive intake of copper can lead to toxicity, which can cause symptoms such as nausea, vomiting, abdominal pain, and liver damage. Long-term exposure to high levels of copper can also result in neurological symptoms such as tremors and cognitive impairment. In extreme cases, copper poisoning can cause liver and kidney damage, hemolytic anemia, and even death.

Acute copper poisoning is rare and typically results from ingesting large amounts of copper-containing substances, such as copper salts or contaminated food and water. Chronic copper toxicity can occur from long-term exposure to elevated levels of copper, for example, from contaminated drinking water.

Contraindications

Individuals with Wilson's disease, a genetic disorder that causes excessive copper accumulation in the body, should not receive copper infusion. In addition, individuals with liver disease or renal failure should be monitored carefully when receiving copper infusion, as these conditions may affect copper metabolism.

Who is a Good Candidate to Receive Copper Infusion

Individuals with copper deficiency, anemia, or other medical conditions that may benefit from copper supplementation may be good candidates for copper infusion.

Is Copper Used with Other Compounds

Copper may be used in conjunction with other compounds in IV therapy, such as amino acids, vitamins, and minerals. The specific combination of compounds used will depend on the individual's medical condition and overall health status.

Frequency of Treatments

The frequency of copper infusion will depend on the individual's specific medical condition and overall health status.

Special Notes

Copper levels can be measured through a blood test, which can help identify copper deficiency or toxicity. It is important to monitor copper levels during copper infusion therapy to prevent potential adverse effects.

Clinical Information

1. What forms does copper come in?
   Copper is available in various forms, including copper gluconate, copper sulfate, and copper oxide. It is also found in many food sources, such as liver, shellfish, nuts, and whole grains.

2. What are the daily dosage limits?
   The recommended daily dosage of copper varies depending on the individual's age, gender, and health status. General daily dosages typically range from 0.9 to 1.3 milligrams per

day for adults, while higher dosages up to 10 milligrams per day may be used in certain cases under medical supervision.

3. How is copper stored?
    Copper supplements should be stored in a cool, dry place, away from direct sunlight and heat. It is important to follow the storage instructions provided by the manufacturer to ensure maximal potency and efficacy.

4. How is copper prepared for IV infusion?
    Copper can be prepared for IV infusion by reconstituting it with sterile water or saline solution. The prepared solution should be used immediately or refrigerated for later use. It is important to use freshly prepared copper solutions for IV infusion to ensure maximal potency and efficacy.

5. Treatment protocols:
    Copper has been studied for its potential therapeutic benefits in various health conditions, including anemia, osteoporosis, and Wilson's disease. However, the optimal dosage and duration of copper supplementation for different health conditions have not been fully established and may vary depending on the individual's needs and response to treatment. For example, for the treatment of anemia, a standard protocol may involve daily doses of 2 milligrams of copper for up to 8 weeks. For the treatment of Wilson's disease, a standard protocol may involve daily doses of up to 4 milligrams of copper for an extended period.

6. What is the half-life of copper?

The half-life of copper in the body varies depending on the dose and the route of administration. In general, the half-life of orally administered copper is relatively short, with a half-life of approximately 12 to 16 hours. The half-life of intravenously administered copper is shorter, with a half-life of approximately 4 to 5 hours.

7. Is it stable?

Copper is a relatively stable compound that is not affected by heat or light. It is highly soluble in water and is not sensitive to moisture. Copper supplements should be stored in a cool, dry place, away from direct sunlight and heat, to ensure maximal potency and efficacy.

References

1. National Institutes of Health. Copper. https://ods.od.nih.gov/factsheets/Copper-HealthProfessional/

2. Klevay LM. Copper. In: Ross AC, Caballero B, Cousins RJ, Tucker KL, Ziegler TR, eds. Modern Nutrition in Health and Disease. 11th ed. Philadelphia, PA: Lippincott Williams & Wilkins; 2012:224-239.

Selenium

Selenium is an essential mineral that has several important roles in the body, including antioxidant activity, thyroid hormone metabolism, and immune system function.

Benefits of Selenium

It acts as a cofactor for various enzymes and proteins that play vital roles in cellular function and homeostasis. Selenium is also involved in the prevention of certain types of cancer and cardiovascular disease.

Dosage recommendations

The recommended dietary allowance (RDA) for selenium is 55 micrograms (mcg) per day for adults. The upper limit for selenium intake is 400 mcg per day. The appropriate dosage of selenium for IV hydration therapy may vary depending on the individual's specific needs and health conditions. It is important to consult with a healthcare provider before starting any supplementation.

Conditions treated with Selenium

Selenium deficiency can lead to a variety of health problems, including muscle weakness, fatigue, and impaired immune function. It may also increase the risk of certain types of cancer, including prostate, lung, and colorectal cancer. IV selenium therapy may be recommended for individuals who are at risk of selenium deficiency or who have certain health conditions that may benefit from increased selenium levels.

Signs of Selenium deficiency

Signs of selenium deficiency may include muscle weakness, fatigue, cognitive decline, and impaired immune function. In severe cases, it may lead to Keshan disease, a type of heart disease that occurs in areas with selenium-poor soils.

Signs of Selenium toxicity

Selenium toxicity is rare but may occur with excessive supplementation. Signs of selenium toxicity may include nausea, vomiting, hair loss, nail brittleness, skin rashes, and nervous system abnormalities. In extreme cases, selenium toxicity can cause severe respiratory and cardiovascular complications, kidney failure, and even death. However, such cases are relatively rare.

Selenium toxicity, also known as selenosis, can occur from ingesting large doses of selenium over a short period of time or from consuming lower doses over an extended period. Symptoms of selenium toxicity can range from mild to severe and may include gastrointestinal issues, hair loss, skin rash, fatigue, irritability, and neurological problems.

To avoid selenium toxicity, it is important to consume selenium within the recommended dietary allowances (RDAs). The RDAs for selenium differ based on age, sex, and life stage, but for adults, the general recommendation is around 55 micrograms per day.

Contraindications

Individuals with selenium allergies or those taking certain medications, such as blood thinners or cholesterol-lowering drugs, should avoid selenium supplementation or IV therapy. High doses of selenium may also be harmful to pregnant women and children.

Who is a good candidate to receive selenium infusion

Selenium infusion may be recommended for individuals who have a deficiency or who require higher levels of selenium due to certain health conditions, such as thyroid disorders, cardiovascular disease, and cancer.

Is selenium used with other compounds

Selenium may be used in combination with other antioxidants, such as vitamin C and vitamin E, to enhance their beneficial effects. It may also be used in combination with other minerals, such as zinc, to support immune function.

Frequency of treatments

The frequency of selenium IV therapy may vary depending on the individual's specific needs and health conditions.

Special Notes

Measuring selenium levels through blood tests may be helpful in identifying individuals who may benefit from IV selenium therapy. It is also important to note that different forms of selenium may have different absorption rates and bioavailability. The most commonly used form of selenium in IV therapy is sodium selenite.

Clinical Information

1. What forms does selenium come in?
   Selenium is an essential trace element that is naturally present in many foods, and is also available in supplement form, such as capsules, tablets, and liquid drops.

2. What are the daily dosage limits?
   The recommended daily allowance of selenium varies by age,

gender, and health status. For adults, the recommended daily intake of selenium is 55 micrograms per day. It is important to not exceed the tolerable upper intake level (UL) of selenium, which is set at 400 micrograms per day for adults.

3. How is selenium stored?
Selenium supplements should be stored in a cool, dry place, away from direct sunlight and heat.

4. How is selenium prepared for IV infusion?
Selenium can be prepared for IV infusion by reconstituting it with sterile water or saline solution. The prepared solution should be used immediately or refrigerated for later use. It is important to use freshly prepared selenium solutions for IV infusion to ensure maximal potency and efficacy.

5. Treatment protocols:
Selenium supplementation has been studied for its potential therapeutic benefits in various health conditions, such as thyroid disease, cancer, and cardiovascular disease. However, the optimal dosage and duration of selenium supplementation for different health conditions have not been fully established and may vary depending on the individual's needs and response to treatment.

6. What is the half-life of selenium?
The half-life of selenium in the body varies depending on the form of selenium and individual metabolism, with an average half-life of around 27-40 hours.

7. Is it stable?

Selenium is a relatively stable compound that is not affected by heat or light. It is highly sensitive to oxidative damage and can be rapidly degraded in the presence of oxygen. Selenium supplements should be stored in a cool, dry place, away from direct sunlight and heat, to ensure maximal potency and efficacy.

References

1. Rayman MP. The importance of selenium to human health. Lancet. 2000; 356(9225):233-241. doi:10.1016/s0140-6736(00)02490-9

2. Kieliszek M, Błażejak S, Blazejak S. Current knowledge on the importance of selenium in food for living organisms: a review. Molecules. 2016;21(5):609. doi:10.3390/molecules21050609

3. Combs GF Jr. Selenium in global food systems. Br J Nutr. 2001;85(5):517-547. doi:10.1079/bjn2000281

Chromium

Chromium is an essential mineral that plays a key role in the metabolism of carbohydrates, lipids, and proteins.

Benefits of Chromium

It is necessary for the proper functioning of insulin, a hormone that regulates blood sugar levels. Chromium has also been shown to have potential benefits for weight management, glucose metabolism, and cardiovascular health.

Dosage recommendations

The recommended daily intake of chromium for adults is 20-35 micrograms per day. In IV hydration, dosages may vary based on the specific treatment plan and the patient's individual needs. It is important to consult with a healthcare provider to determine the appropriate dosage for IV administration.

Conditions treated with Chromium

Chromium supplementation may be beneficial for individuals with insulin resistance, type 2 diabetes, metabolic syndrome, and other conditions related to blood sugar regulation. Additionally, chromium has been studied for its potential effects on weight loss, athletic performance, and cognitive function.

Signs of Chromium deficiency

Signs of chromium deficiency may include impaired glucose tolerance, insulin resistance, elevated blood sugar levels, and increased risk of diabetes. Other potential symptoms may include fatigue, irritability, and weight gain.

Signs of Chromium toxicity

Excessive intake of chromium supplements may lead to toxicity and potential adverse effects, including gastrointestinal issues, skin reactions, and liver and kidney damage. In severe cases of chromium poisoning, organ failure or other complications can lead to death. However, such cases are relatively rare and usually associated with industrial accidents or environmental contamination.

Excessive intake of chromium can lead to chromium toxicity, which can be harmful and potentially life-threatening in severe cases. The risk of toxicity is generally associated with the ingestion of large amounts of inorganic hexavalent chromium (Cr(VI)), which is highly toxic and can be found in industrial settings and certain contaminated water supplies.

Contraindications

Individuals with liver or kidney disease or those taking certain medications, such as antacids or corticosteroids, may be at an increased risk of adverse effects from chromium supplementation. It is important to consult with a healthcare provider before starting any new supplement regimen.

Who is a good candidate to receive Chromium infusion

Individuals with specific medical conditions or those with a known deficiency in chromium may be good candidates for IV infusion of chromium. It is important to consult with a healthcare provider to determine if IV administration is appropriate and necessary.

Is Chromium used with other compounds

Chromium may be used in combination with other nutrients and compounds for IV administration, such as B vitamins and amino acids, depending on the specific treatment plan.

Frequency of treatments

The frequency of IV administration of chromium may vary depending on the individual's needs and treatment plan. It is important to consult with a healthcare provider to determine the appropriate frequency of IV administration.

Special Notes

Measuring chromium levels in the body is not routinely performed, as there is no widely accepted method for measuring chromium status. However, individuals with specific medical conditions or those with a known deficiency in chromium may benefit from testing to determine their chromium levels.

Clinical Information

1. What forms does chromium come in?
   Chromium is an essential mineral that is available in supplement form, such as capsules, tablets, and liquid drops. It is also present in small amounts in certain foods, such as broccoli, grape juice, and whole grains.

2. What are the daily dosage limits?
   The recommended daily intake of chromium varies by age, gender, and health status. For adults, the recommended daily intake of chromium is 20-35 micrograms per day. It is important to not exceed the tolerable upper intake level (UL) of chromium, which is set at 1000 micrograms per day for adults.

3. How is chromium stored?
   Chromium supplements should be stored in a cool, dry place, away from direct sunlight and heat.

4. How is chromium prepared for IV infusion?

Chromium can be prepared for IV infusion by reconstituting it with sterile water or saline solution. The prepared solution should be used immediately or refrigerated for later use. It is important to use freshly prepared chromium solutions for IV infusion to ensure maximal potency and efficacy.

5. Treatment protocols:

Chromium supplementation has been studied for its potential therapeutic benefits in various health conditions, such as type 2 diabetes and metabolic syndrome. However, the optimal dosage and duration of chromium supplementation for different health conditions have not been fully established and may vary depending on the individual's needs and response to treatment.

6. What is the half-life of chromium?

The half-life of chromium in the body varies depending on the form of chromium and individual metabolism, with an average half-life of around 24-48 hours.

7. Is it stable?

Chromium is a relatively stable compound that is not affected by heat or light. It is highly sensitive to oxidative damage and can be rapidly degraded in the presence of oxygen. Chromium supplements should be stored in a cool, dry place, away from direct sunlight and heat, to ensure maximal potency and efficacy.

References

1. Anderson RA. Chromium and polyphenols from cinnamon improve insulin sensitivity. Proc Nutr Soc. 2008 Feb;67(1):48-53.

2. Bailey RL, et al. Dietary supplement use in the United States, 2003-2006. J Nutr. 2011 Feb;141(2):261-6.

3. Vincent JB. The potential value and toxicity of chromium picolinate as a nutritional supplement, weight loss agent and muscle development agent. Sports Med. 2003;33(3):213-30.

Conclusion

Minerals play a crucial role in maintaining the body's overall health and well-being, making their inclusion in IV hydration therapy an essential consideration. The proper balance of these vital elements, including calcium, magnesium, zinc, chromium, copper, and selenium, can significantly impact a person's recovery, performance, and general health. However, it is critical to administer these minerals at safe and appropriate doses to avoid the risk of toxicity or imbalances. Healthcare professionals must carefully evaluate individual patient needs and closely monitor for any potential side effects or complications. By understanding the role and significance of each mineral, practitioners can create customized IV hydration treatments that effectively address deficiencies, enhance recovery, and promote optimal health for their patients.

CHAPTER 5 - AMINO ACIDS

Amino acids are the building blocks of proteins, which are essential for the growth and repair of tissues in the body. There are 20 different types of amino acids, and they can be classified as essential or nonessential.

Essential amino acids cannot be produced by the body and must be obtained through the diet or supplements, while nonessential amino acids can be produced by the body. Amino acids play a crucial role in many physiological processes, including muscle growth and repair, immune function, and energy production.

The nine essential amino acids are:

1. Histidine: Histidine is important for the growth and repair of tissues and plays a role in the production of red and white blood cells.

2. Isoleucine: Isoleucine is involved in the regulation of blood sugar levels and the production of hemoglobin.

3. Leucine: Leucine is important for muscle growth and repair, and is also involved in the regulation of blood sugar levels.

4. Lysine: Lysine is important for the synthesis of collagen and other proteins, as well as for the absorption of calcium and the production of carnitine.

5. Methionine: Methionine is a precursor for other amino acids and is involved in the production of proteins, as well as in the metabolism of fats and other nutrients.

6. Phenylalanine: Phenylalanine is involved in the production of other amino acids and neurotransmitters, including dopamine and norepinephrine.

7. Threonine: Threonine is involved in the production of collagen, elastin, and other proteins, as well as in the metabolism of fats and immune function.

8. Tryptophan: Tryptophan is a precursor for the neurotransmitter serotonin and is also involved in the synthesis of niacin.

9. Valine: Valine is important for muscle growth and repair, as well as for the regulation of blood sugar levels.

There are 11 nonessential amino acids Nonessential amino acids are amino acids that can be synthesized by the body and therefore do not need to be obtained from the diet. The body can produce nonessential amino acids by breaking down dietary proteins or by synthesizing them from other amino acids or precursor molecules. However, in certain situations such as illness, injury, or intense exercise, the body may not be able to produce enough nonessential amino acids to meet its needs, and supplementation may be necessary.

1. Alanine: Alanine is important for glucose metabolism and energy production.

2. Arginine: Arginine is involved in the synthesis of nitric oxide, which helps to dilate blood vessels and improve blood flow. It also plays a role in wound healing and immune function.

3. Asparagine: Asparagine is involved in the synthesis of proteins and nucleotides.

4. Aspartic acid: Aspartic acid is involved in the synthesis of other amino acids and plays a role in energy production.

5. Cysteine: Cysteine is important for the formation of proteins and is also involved in the synthesis of glutathione, a powerful antioxidant.

6. Glutamic acid: Glutamic acid is involved in the synthesis of other amino acids and plays a role in energy production.

7. Glutamine: Glutamine is important for immune function and gut health. It is also involved in the synthesis of proteins and nucleotides.

8. Glycine: Glycine is involved in the synthesis of proteins and is also an important neurotransmitter in the central nervous system.

9. Proline: Proline is important for collagen synthesis, which is essential for healthy skin, joints, and connective tissue.

10. Serine: Serine is involved in the synthesis of proteins and nucleotides, as well as the metabolism of fats and fatty acids.

11. Tyrosine: Tyrosine is involved in the production of several important neurotransmitters, including dopamine, norepinephrine, and epinephrine. It is also involved in the synthesis of thyroid hormones.

Nonessential amino acids are not typically supplemented in IV hydration clinics. Instead, IV hydration formulas typically focus on essential amino acids, which are amino acids that the body cannot produce and must obtain from the diet or supplements.

However, some nonessential amino acids may be present in small amounts in IV hydration formulas, as they play important roles in various metabolic processes in the body. For example, the nonessential amino acid glycine is sometimes included in IV hydration formulas due to its role in collagen synthesis and wound healing.

Another nonessential amino acid, alanine, may be included in IV hydration formulas to help promote healthy blood sugar levels.

Glutamine is an amino acid that is involved in many metabolic processes in the body, including the synthesis of proteins, the production of energy, and the regulation of immune function. It is particularly important for maintaining healthy muscle tissue, as it is the most abundant amino acid in muscle tissue. During times of stress or illness, the body's demand for glutamine may increase, and supplementation with IV glutamine may be beneficial.

IV glutamine can help to support muscle recovery and reduce muscle breakdown, particularly in athletes and individuals undergoing intense exercise or training. It may be useful for individuals with gastrointestinal issues, as it can help to support healthy gut function and reduce intestinal inflammation.

Several other amino acids or amino acid combinations worth mentioning are glutathione, L-taurine, L-carnitine, L-citrulline and L-orthinine. The "L" before the name of an amino acid, such as "L-citrulline," indicates the stereochemistry of the amino acid. Stereochemistry refers to the three-dimensional arrangement of atoms in a molecule. In the case of amino acids, the "L" form is the one that is used to build proteins in the body, while the "D" form is rarely found in nature and is not used in protein synthesis. Therefore, when a supplement or medication contains an amino acid with an "L" prefix, it means that the product contains the same form of the amino acid that is found in the human body and is used to build proteins.

Glutathione, taurine, carnitine, citrulline, ornithine, and NAC are a group of compounds referred to as amino acid derivatives. These are molecules that are structurally related to amino acids, but that have been modified in some way. These modifications can include the addition of functional groups, the removal of amino or carboxyl groups, or changes in the side chain structure. Some examples of amino acid derivatives include:

1. Glutathione is a powerful antioxidant that is derived from the amino acids cysteine, glutamic acid, and glycine

2. Taurine is derived from two sulfur-containing amino acids, cysteine and methionine, and is structurally similar to other amino acids. However, unlike other amino acids, taurine does not have a carboxyl group at the end of its molecule, which means it is not incorporated into proteins. Instead, taurine is found in many tissues throughout the body, particularly in the brain, heart, and muscles. It plays important roles in a variety of physiological processes, including the regulation of electrolytes, the modulation of neurotransmitters, and the maintenance of cell membrane stability.

3. Carnitine is an amino acid derivative that is synthesized from the amino acids lysine and methionine, and is involved in the transport of fatty acids into the mitochondria for energy production.

4. Orthinine is produced from the amino acid arginine through a process called decarboxylation, which involves the removal of a carboxyl group from the amino acid. Ornithine plays an important role in the urea cycle, which is responsible for the detoxification of ammonia in the liver. It is also involved in the synthesis of other important molecules, including polyamines and proline.

5. Citrulline is produced from the amino acid ornithine through a process called the urea cycle, which takes place in the liver. Citrulline is involved in the removal of toxic ammonia from the body and the production of nitric oxide, a molecule that helps to dilate blood vessels and improve blood flow. Citrulline is also used as a dietary supplement to improve athletic performance, reduce muscle fatigue and soreness, and support cardiovascular health.

6. N-acetylcysteine (NAC) is a derivative of the naturally occurring amino acid cysteine, and it serves as a precursor to glutathione.

WHY SUPPLEMENT WITH A DERIVATIVE INSTEAD OF THE SOURCE?

There are several reasons why we might choose to supplement with amino acid derivatives rather than the actual amino acid:

1. Increased bioavailability: In some cases, amino acid derivatives may be more readily absorbed and utilized by the body than the actual amino acid. This can be due to differences in molecular structure, solubility, or other factors that affect how the substance is metabolized.

2. Specific health benefits: Some amino acid derivatives have unique health benefits that are not found in the actual amino acid. For example, taurine, a derivative of cysteine and methionine, has been shown to have antioxidant properties and may help to regulate blood pressure and support healthy heart function.

3. Lower toxicity: In some cases, amino acid derivatives may be less toxic or have fewer side effects than the actual amino acid. For example, the oral supplement N-acetylcysteine (NAC) is a derivative of the amino acid cysteine and is commonly used to support liver function and promote respiratory health. NAC is generally considered safe and well-tolerated, even at high doses. NAC is not generally given intravenously.

4. Overall, the decision to supplement with an amino acid derivative versus the actual amino acid will depend on a variety of factors, including the individual's health status, dietary intake, and specific health goals.

In this chapter we will discuss the following amino acids and derivatives due to their practicality in IV hydration.

The most commonly used essential amino acids in IV hydration include:

1. Histidine: Histidine is sometimes included in IV solutions for its potential anti-inflammatory and antioxidant effects.

2. Leucine: Leucine is often included in IV solutions for its potential muscle-building and repair effects.

3. Lysine: Lysine may be included in IV solutions for its potential immune-boosting effects.

4. Methionine: Methionine is sometimes included in IV solutions for its potential detoxifying effects.

5. Threonine: Threonine may be included in IV solutions for its potential immune-boosting effects.

6. Tryptophan: Tryptophan is sometimes included in IV solutions for its potential mood-boosting effects.

7. Valine: Valine is often included in IV solutions for its potential muscle-building and repair effects.

The most commonly used nonessential amino acids in IV hydration include:

1. Alanine:Alanine helps promote healthy blood sugar levels.

2. Arginine:Arginine helps promote circulation and is beneficial for people with high blood pressure or other cardiovascular issues.

3. Glutamine:Glutamine is used in the production of energy, muscle recovery and regulation of the immune system.

4. Glycine:Glycine is used due to its role in collagen synthesis and wound healing.

The most commonly used amino acid derivatives in IV hydration include:

1. Glutathione

2. Taurine

3. Carnitine

4. Orthinine

5. Citrulline

6. NAC

ESSENTIAL AMINO ACIDS IN IV HYDRATION

Histidine

Histidine is a semi-essential amino acid that plays an important role in many physiological processes in the body. While histidine is not commonly used as the primary component of IV hydration solutions, it can be added to these solutions to provide additional nutritional support in certain situations.

Benefits of Histidine

Histidine is involved in many physiological processes in the body, including the production of histamine, a compound that is involved in immune response and inflammation. Histidine also plays a role in the regulation of pH balance in the body, and is involved in the production of red and white blood cells. Additionally, histidine may have antioxidant properties and may help to support wound healing.

Dosage Recommendations

The appropriate dosage of histidine for IV infusion will depend on the specific needs of the patient and the goals of the therapy. However, typical dosages range from 2-4 grams per day for adults. It's important to note that excessive doses of histidine may be toxic.

Conditions Treated with Histidine

While histidine is not commonly used as a standalone therapy for any specific medical condition, it may be added to IV hydration solutions to provide additional nutritional support in certain situations. For example, histidine may be included in IV solutions for patients who are malnourished or who have a condition that affects their ability to absorb nutrients from food.

Signs of Histidine Deficiency

Histidine deficiency is rare, as the body can produce histidine naturally However, in some cases, such as in patients with certain genetic disorders, histidine deficiency may occur. Symptoms of histidine deficiency may include anemia, poor wound healing, and fatigue.

Signs of Histidine Toxicity

Excessive doses of histidine may be toxic and may cause symptoms such as headaches, nausea, and vomiting.

Contraindications

Histidine should be used with caution in patients with liver or kidney disease, as these organs are responsible for metabolizing amino acids. Additionally, histidine should be used with caution in patients with a history of allergies or asthma, as it may exacerbate these conditions.

Who is a Good Candidate to Receive Histidine Infusion?

Patients who are malnourished or who have a condition that affects their ability to absorb nutrients from food may be good candidates to receive histidine infusion. Additionally, patients who have a condition that affects their immune system or who are recovering from an injury or surgery may benefit from histidine infusion as part of a broader IV hydration solution.

Is Histidine Used with Other Compounds or Amino Acids?

Histidine may be used in combination with other compounds and amino acids in IV hydration solutions. For example, it may be combined with other essential amino acids, such as leucine, isoleucine, and valine, to provide additional nutritional support.

Frequency of Treatments

The frequency of histidine infusion will depend on the specific needs of the patient and the goals of the therapy. However, typical dosages range from 2-4 grams per day for adults, and the infusion may be given daily or several times per week, depending on the patient's needs.

Special Notes

In addition to IV hydration solutions, histidine may be added to certain food products as a natural flavor enhancer. Histidine has a slightly sweet and savory taste and can help to improve the overall flavor of foods.

Clinical Information

1. What forms does histidine come in?
   Histidine is an essential amino acid that is found in protein-rich foods such as meat, fish, and dairy products. Histidine supplements are also available in various forms, including capsules, tablets, powders, and liquid forms.

2. What are the daily dosage limits?
   There is no established daily dosage limit for histidine, as it is an essential amino acid that the body requires for normal growth and development.

3. How is histidine stored?
   Histidine supplements should be stored in a cool, dry place, away from direct sunlight and heat.

4. How is histidine prepared for IV infusion?
   Histidine can be prepared for IV infusion by reconstituting it with sterile water or saline solution. The prepared solution should be used immediately or refrigerated for later use. It is important to use freshly prepared histidine solutions for IV infusion to ensure maximal potency and efficacy.

5. Treatment protocols:

Histidine has been studied for its potential therapeutic benefits in various health conditions, including rheumatoid arthritis and anemia. However, the optimal dosage and duration of histidine supplementation for different health conditions have not been fully established and may vary depending on the individual's needs and response to treatment. For example, for the treatment of rheumatoid arthritis, a standard protocol may involve daily doses of 2 grams of histidine for up to 12 weeks. For the treatment of anemia, a protocol may involve daily doses of 15-25 milligrams of histidine per kilogram of body weight for up to 8 weeks.

6. What is the half-life of histidine?

The half-life of histidine in the body is relatively short - approximately 2-3 hours. This short half-life means that histidine levels can decline rapidly under conditions of high oxidative stress or toxin exposure.

7. Is it stable?

Histidine is a relatively stable compound that is not affected by heat, light, or air. However, histidine supplements should be stored in a cool, dry place, away from direct sunlight and heat, to ensure maximal potency and efficacy.

References

1. Wu G. Amino acids: metabolism, functions, and nutrition. Amino Acids. 2009;37(1):1-17. doi: 10.1007/s00726-009-0269-0. PMID: 19301095.

2. Mehta NM, Corkins MR, Lyman B, et al. Defining pediatric malnutrition: a paradigm shift toward etiology-related definitions. JPEN J Parenter Enteral Nutr. 2013;37(4):460-481. doi: 10.1177/0148607113487664. PMID: 23620359.

3. Marik PE, Hooper MH. Doctor, is this IV really necessary? N Engl J Med. 2018;379(8):769-771. doi: 10.1056/NEJMp1805820. PMID: 30110597.

4. Deutz NE, Safar A, Schutzler S, et al. Muscle protein synthesis in cancer patients can be stimulated with a specially formulated medical food. Clin Nutr. 2011;30(6):759-768. doi: 10.1016/j.clnu.2011.06.007. PMID: 21775114.

5. Schulman RC, Mechanick JI. Metabolic and nutritional support in the critically ill: why bother?. Curr Opin Crit Care. 2007;13(2):170-176. doi: 10.1097/MCC.0b013e3280142675. PMID: 17327775.

Leucine

Leucine is an essential amino acid that plays a crucial role in protein synthesis and muscle maintenance. While leucine is not commonly used as the primary component of IV hydration solutions, it can be added to these solutions to provide additional nutritional support in certain situations.

Benefits of Leucine

Leucine is a branched-chain amino acid (BCAA) that is involved in protein synthesis and muscle maintenance. Leucine has been shown to promote muscle protein synthesis, which can help to improve muscle growth and recovery after exercise. Leucine may also have anti-inflammatory properties and may help to improve insulin sensitivity, which can be beneficial for patients with type 2 diabetes.

Dosage Recommendations

The appropriate dosage of leucine for IV infusion will depend on the specific needs of the patient and the goals of the therapy. However, typical dosages range from 4-8 grams per day for adults. It's important to note that excessive doses of leucine may be toxic.

Conditions Treated with Leucine

While leucine is not commonly used as a standalone therapy for any specific medical condition, it may be added to IV hydration solutions to provide additional nutritional support in certain situations. For example, leucine may be included in IV solutions for patients who are malnourished or who have a condition that affects their ability to absorb nutrients from food.

Signs of Leucine Deficiency

Leucine deficiency is rare, as the body requires this amino acid to function properly. However, in some cases, such as in patients with certain genetic disorders, leucine deficiency may occur. Symptoms of leucine deficiency may include muscle weakness, fatigue, and poor wound healing.

Signs of Leucine Toxicity

Excessive doses of leucine may be toxic and may cause symptoms such as nausea, vomiting, and diarrhea. It's important to follow the guidance of a qualified healthcare professional when administering leucine to avoid the risk of toxicity.

Contraindications

Leucine should be used with caution in patients with liver or kidney disease, as these organs are responsible for metabolizing amino acids. Additionally, leucine should be used with caution in patients who are allergic to peanuts or soy, as these foods are rich in leucine.

Who is a Good Candidate to Receive Leucine Infusion?

Patients who are malnourished or who have a condition that affects their ability to absorb nutrients from food may be good candidates to receive leucine infusion. Additionally, athletes who are looking to improve muscle growth and recovery may benefit from leucine infusion as part of a broader IV hydration solution.

Is Leucine Used with Other Compounds or Amino Acids?

Leucine may be used in combination with other compounds and amino acids in IV hydration solutions. For example, it may be combined with other BCAAs, such as isoleucine and valine, to provide additional nutritional and athletic performance support.

Frequency of Treatments

The frequency of leucine infusion will depend on the specific needs of the patient and the goals of the therapy. However, typical dosages range from 4-8 grams per day for adults, and the infusion may be given daily or several times per week, depending on the patient's needs.

Clinical Information

1. What forms does leucine come in?

    Leucine is an essential branched-chain amino acid that is found in protein-rich foods such as meat, eggs, and dairy products. Leucine supplements are also available in various forms, including capsules, tablets, powders, and liquid forms.

2. What are the daily dosage limits?

    There is no established daily dosage limit for leucine, as it is an essential amino acid that the body requires for normal growth and development.

3. How is leucine stored?

    Leucine supplements should be stored in a cool, dry place, away from direct sunlight and heat.

4. How is leucine prepared for IV infusion?

    Leucine can be prepared for IV infusion by reconstituting it with sterile water or saline solution. The prepared solution should be used immediately or refrigerated for later use. It is important to use freshly prepared leucine solutions for IV infusion to ensure maximal potency and efficacy.

5. Treatment protocols:

    Leucine has been studied for its potential therapeutic benefits in various health conditions, including muscle wasting, diabetes, and neurological disorders. However, the optimal dosage and duration of leucine supplementation for different health conditions have not been fully established and may vary depending on the individual's needs and response to treatment. For example, for the treatment of muscle wasting, a standard protocol may involve daily doses of 10-15 grams of leucine for up to 12 weeks. For the treatment of diabetes, a protocol may involve daily doses of 5 grams of leucine for up to 8 weeks.

6. What is the half-life of leucine?

The half-life of leucine in the body is relatively short - approximately 1-2 hours. This short half-life means that leucine levels can decline rapidly under conditions of high oxidative stress or toxin exposure.

7. Is it stable?

Leucine is a relatively stable compound that is not affected by heat, light, or air. However, leucine supplements should be stored in a cool, dry place, away from direct sunlight and heat, to ensure maximal potency and efficacy.

References

1. Norton LE, Layman DK. Leucine regulates translation initiation of protein synthesis in skeletal muscle after exercise. J Nutr. 2006;136(2):533S-537S. doi: 10.1093/jn/136.2.533S. PMID: 16424141.

2. Deutz NE, Safar A, Schutzler S, et al. Muscle protein synthesis in cancer patients can be stimulated with a specially formulated medical food. Clin Nutr. 2011;30(6):759-768. doi: 10.1016/j.clnu.2011.06.007. PMID: 21775114.

3. Biolo G, Tipton KD, Klein S, Wolfe RR. An abundant supply of amino acids enhances the metabolic effect of exercise on muscle protein. Am J Physiol. 1997;273(1 Pt 1):E122-9. doi: 10.1152/ajpendo.1997.273.1.E122. PMID: 9252488.

4. Gualano AB, Bozza T, Lopes De Campos P, et al. Branched-chain amino acids supplementation enhances exercise capacity and lipid oxidation during endurance exercise after muscle glycogen depletion. J Sports Med Phys Fitness. 2011;51(1):82-8. PMID: 21297567.

5. Macotela Y, Emanuelli B, Bang AM, et al. Dietary leucine--an environmental modifier of insulin resistance acting on multiple levels of metabolism. PLoS One. 2011;6(6):e21187. doi: 10.1371/journal.pone.0021187. PMID: 21695119.

Lysine

Lysine is an essential amino acid that plays an important role in protein synthesis and immune function. While lysine is not commonly used as the primary component of IV hydration solutions, it can be added to these solutions to provide additional nutritional support in certain situations.

Benefits of Lysine

Lysine is involved in many physiological processes in the body, including the production of enzymes and hormones, the formation of collagen and other proteins, and the regulation of immune function. Lysine may also have antiviral properties and may help to reduce the severity and duration of cold sores caused by the herpes simplex virus.

Dosage Recommendations

The appropriate dosage of lysine for IV infusion will depend on the specific needs of the patient and the goals of the therapy. However, typical dosages range from 2-4 grams per day for adults. It's important to note that excessive doses of lysine may be toxic.

Conditions Treated with Lysine

While lysine is not commonly used as a standalone therapy for any specific medical condition, it may be added to IV hydration solutions to provide additional nutritional support in certain situations. For example, lysine may be included in IV solutions for patients who are malnourished or who have a condition that affects their ability to absorb nutrients from food.

Signs of Lysine Deficiency

Lysine deficiency is rare, as the body requires this amino acid to function properly. However, in some cases, such as in patients with certain genetic disorders, lysine deficiency may occur. Symptoms of lysine deficiency may include fatigue, anemia, and decreased appetite.

Signs of Lysine Toxicity

Excessive doses of lysine may be toxic and may cause symptoms such as nausea, vomiting, and diarrhea.

Contraindications

Lysine should be used with caution in patients with liver or kidney disease, as these organs are responsible for metabolizing amino acids.

Additionally, lysine should be used with caution in patients who are allergic to lysine or who have a history of kidney stones.

Who is a Good Candidate to Receive Lysine Infusion?

Patients who are malnourished or who have a condition that affects their ability to absorb nutrients from food may be good candidates to receive lysine infusion. Additionally, patients who have a condition that affects their immune system or who are recovering from an injury or surgery may benefit from lysine infusion as part of a broader IV hydration solution.

Is Lysine Used with Other Compounds or Amino Acids?

Lysine may be used in combination with other compounds and amino acids in IV hydration solutions. For example, it may be combined with other essential amino acids, such as leucine and valine, to provide additional nutritional support.

Frequency of Treatments

The frequency of lysine infusion will depend on the specific needs of the patient and the goals of the therapy. However, typical dosages range from 2-4 grams per day for adults, and the infusion may be given daily or several times per week, depending on the patient's needs.

Clinical Information

1. What forms does lysine come in?

    Lysine is an essential amino acid that is found in protein-rich foods such as meat, fish, and dairy products. Lysine supplements are also available in various forms, including capsules, tablets, powders, and liquid forms.

2. What are the daily dosage limits?
There is no established daily dosage limit for lysine, as it is an essential amino acid that the body requires for normal growth and development.

3. How is lysine stored?
Lysine supplements should be stored in a cool, dry place, away from direct sunlight and heat.

4. How is lysine prepared for IV infusion?
Lysine can be prepared for IV infusion by reconstituting it with sterile water or saline solution. The prepared solution should be used immediately or refrigerated for later use. It is important to use freshly prepared lysine solutions for IV infusion to ensure maximal potency and efficacy.

5. Treatment protocols:
Lysine has been studied for its potential therapeutic benefits in various health conditions, including herpes infections, osteoporosis, and anxiety. However, the optimal dosage and duration of lysine supplementation for different health conditions have not been fully established and may vary depending on the individual's needs and response to treatment. For example, for the treatment of herpes infections, a standard protocol may involve daily doses of 1-3 grams of lysine for up to 6 months. For the treatment of osteoporosis, a

protocol may involve daily doses of 1.5 grams of lysine for up to 24 months.

6. What is the half-life of lysine?

The half-life of lysine in the body is relatively short - approximately 1-2 hours. This short half-life means that lysine levels can decline rapidly under conditions of high oxidative stress or toxin exposure.

7. Is it stable?

Lysine is a relatively stable compound that is not affected by heat, light, or air. However, lysine supplements should be stored in a cool, dry place, away from direct sunlight and heat, to ensure maximal potency and efficacy.

References

1. Smriga M, Ando T, Akutsu M. Effect of L-lysine hydrochloride on the recovery of fatigue sensation after heavy-load squat exercise. Eur J Appl Physiol. 2007;100(3):385-390. doi: 10.1007/s00421-007-0443-3. PMID: 17345062.

2. 2. Liu T, Peng YF, Jia C, et al. Lysine regulates glucose metabolism via promotion of insulin secretion and suppression of pyruvate kinase activity in pancreatic β-cells. Food Funct. 2017;8(11):4064-4072. doi: 10.1039/ c7fo01161h. PMID: 28956038.

3. Trovato A, Nuhlicek DN, Midtling JE, et al. Lysine supplementation during total parenteral nutrition prevents

depletion of free l-arginine. J Parenter Enteral Nutr. 1996;20(3):217-222. doi: 10.1177/0148607196020003217. PMID: 8690234.

4. Li W, Li X, Li T, et al. Effect of lysine supplementation on health and growth of grass carp (Ctenopharyngodon idella) under intensive farming. Fish Shellfish Immunol. 2014;39(1):147-155. doi: 10.1016/j.fsi.2014.04.024. PMID: 24793441.

5. Rezaei R, Wu Z, Hou Y, et al. Amino acids and immune function. Br J Nutr. 2013;110(8):1542-1559. doi: 10.1017/S0007114513001019. PMID: 23551944.

Methionine

Methionine is an essential amino acid that plays a vital role in protein synthesis, detoxification, and the formation of important molecules such as glutathione. While methionine is not commonly used as the primary component of IV hydration solutions, it can be added to these solutions to provide additional nutritional support in certain situations.

Benefits of Methionine

Methionine is involved in many important processes in the body, including the synthesis of proteins, DNA, and other molecules, as well as the regulation of gene expression. Methionine also plays a crucial role in the production of glutathione, which is an important antioxidant and detoxifying molecule. Methionine may also have anti-inflammatory properties and may help to improve liver function.

Dosage Recommendations

The appropriate dosage of methionine for IV infusion will depend on the specific needs of the patient and the goals of the therapy. However, typical dosages range from 1-2 grams per day for adults. It's important to note that excessive doses of methionine may be toxic.

Conditions Treated with Methionine

While methionine is not commonly used as a standalone therapy for any specific medical condition, it may be added to IV hydration solutions to provide additional nutritional support in certain situations. For example, methionine may be included in IV solutions for patients who are malnourished or who have a condition that affects their ability to absorb nutrients from food.

Signs of Methionine Deficiency

Methionine deficiency is rare, as the body requires this amino acid to function properly. However, in some cases, such as in patients with certain genetic disorders, methionine deficiency may occur. Symptoms of methionine deficiency may include fatigue, muscle weakness, and decreased immunity.

Signs of Methionine Toxicity

Excessive doses of methionine may be toxic and may cause symptoms such as nausea, vomiting, and diarrhea.

Contraindications

Methionine should be used with caution in patients with liver or kidney disease, as these organs are responsible for metabolizing amino acids. Additionally, methionine should be used with caution in patients who have a history of peptic ulcer disease or who are taking certain medications, such as anti-inflammatory drugs.

People with sulfur allergies may be allergic to certain forms of sulfur, such as sulfites, which are commonly found in foods and beverages. However, methionine is not a sulfite and does not contain the same type of sulfur molecule that may trigger an allergic reaction.

Methionine contains sulfur atoms, but they are in the form of sulfhydryl (-SH) groups, which are not typically associated with sulfur allergies.

Regardless, individuals with a history of sulfur allergies or sensitivities should still discuss the use of methionine before use, as they may have individual factors that make them more susceptible to allergic reactions.

Who is a Good Candidate to Receive Methionine Infusion?

Patients who are malnourished or who have a condition that affects their ability to absorb nutrients from food may be good candidates to receive methionine infusion. Additionally, patients who have a condition that affects their liver or who are recovering from an injury or surgery may benefit from methionine infusion as part of a broader IV hydration solution.

Is Methionine Used with Other Compounds or Amino Acids?

Methionine may be used in combination with other compounds and amino acids in IV hydration solutions. For example, it may be combined with other essential amino acids, such as leucine and valine, to provide additional nutritional support.

Frequency of Treatments

The frequency of methionine infusion will depend on the specific needs of the patient and the goals of the therapy. However, typical dosages range from 1-2 grams per day for adults, and the infusion may be given daily or several times per week, depending on the patient's needs.

Special Notes

Methionine is sensitive to light and can degrade when exposed to it. This is because the sulfur-containing amino acid residues in methionine can be oxidized when exposed to light, leading to a decrease in the activity of the molecule.

To protect against light-induced degradation, methionine should be stored in a cool, dry, and dark place. IV methionine solutions should be stored in a light-resistant container or covered with a light-proof wrap during administration to prevent exposure to light.

Clinical Information

1. What forms does methionine come in?
   Methionine is an essential amino acid that is found in protein-rich foods such as meat, fish, and dairy products. Methionine supplements are also available in various forms, including capsules, tablets, powders, and liquid forms.

2. What are the daily dosage limits?
   There is no established daily dosage limit for methionine, as

it is an essential amino acid that the body requires for normal growth and development.

3. How is methionine stored?

Methionine supplements should be stored in a cool, dry, and darkplace, away from light and heat.

4. How is methionine prepared for IV infusion?

Methionine can be prepared for IV infusion by reconstituting it with sterile water or saline solution. The prepared solution should be used immediately or refrigerated for later use. As noted above, it should be stored in a light-resistant container or covered with a light-proof wrap during administration. It is important to use freshly prepared methionine solutions for IV infusion to ensure maximal potency and efficacy.

5. Treatment protocols:

Methionine has been studied for its potential therapeutic benefits in various health conditions, including liver disease, depression, and cancer. However, the optimal dosage and duration of methionine supplementation for different health conditions have not been fully established and may vary depending on the individual's needs and response to treatment. For example, for the treatment of liver disease, a standard protocol may involve daily doses of 500 milligrams to 1 gram of methionine for up to 6 months. For the treatment of depression, a protocol may involve daily doses of 500 milligrams to 1 gram of methionine for up to 12 weeks.

6. What is the half-life of methionine?

The half-life of methionine in the body is relatively short -

approximately 3-4 hours. This short half-life means that methionine levels can decline rapidly under conditions of high oxidative stress or toxin exposure.

7. Is it stable?
Methionine is a compound that is not affected by heat but can be easily degraded by light-exposure. See above to storage and handling recommendations

References

1. Stipanuk MH, Caudill MA. Biochemical, Physiological, and Molecular Aspects of Human Nutrition. 4th ed. St. Louis, MO: Saunders/Elsevier; 2013.

2. Mato JM, Martínez-Chantar ML, Lu SC. Methionine metabolism and liver disease. Annu Rev Nutr. 2008;28:273-293. doi: 10.1146/annurev.nutr.28.061807.155424. PMID: 18429680.

3. Du J, Cieslak JA, Welsh JL, et al. Pharmacological manipulation of methionine metabolism in growing mice: A metabolic link between N-acetylcysteine and creatine synthesis. Am J Physiol Endocrinol Metab. 2014;306(10):E1135-E1147. doi: 10.1152/ajpendo.00020.2014. PMID: 24691008.

4. Fan C, Zhang Y, Wang Q, et al. Methionine deprivation suppresses triple-negative breast cancer metastasis in vitro and in vivo. Oncotarget. 2017;8(19):31627-31639. doi: 10.18632/oncotarget.16095. PMID: 28423623.

5. Wu G, Fang YZ, Yang S, Lupton JR, Turner ND. Glutathione metabolism and its implications for health. J Nutr.

2004;134(3):489-492. doi: 10.1093/jn/134.3.489. PMID: 14988435.

Threonine

Threonine is an essential amino acid that plays an important role in protein synthesis and immune function. While threonine is not commonly used as the primary component of IV hydration solutions, it can be added to these solutions to provide additional nutritional support in certain situations.

Benefits of Threonine

Threonine is involved in many physiological processes in the body, including the production of enzymes and hormones, the formation of collagen and other proteins, and the regulation of immune function. Threonine may also have a positive impact on gut health and may help to improve digestion.

Dosage Recommendations

The appropriate dosage of threonine for IV infusion will depend on the specific needs of the patient and the goals of the therapy. However, typical dosages range from 1-2 grams per day for adults. It's important to note that excessive doses of threonine may be toxic.

Conditions Treated with Threonine

While threonine is not commonly used as a standalone therapy for any specific medical condition, it may be added to IV hydration solutions to provide additional nutritional support in certain situations. For example, threonine may be included in IV solutions for patients who are malnourished or who have a condition that affects their ability to absorb nutrients from food.

Signs of Threonine Deficiency

Threonine deficiency is rare, as the body requires this amino acid to function properly. However, in some cases, such as in patients with certain genetic disorders or who are on a severely restricted diet, threonine deficiency may occur. Symptoms of threonine deficiency may include fatigue, irritability, and decreased immunity.

Signs of Threonine Toxicity

Excessive doses of threonine may be toxic and may cause symptoms such as nausea, vomiting, and diarrhea.

Contraindications

Threonine should be used with caution in patients with liver or kidney disease, as these organs are responsible for metabolizing amino acids. Additionally, threonine should be used with caution in patients who are allergic to threonine or who have a history of kidney stones.

Who is a Good Candidate to Receive Threonine Infusion?

Patients who are malnourished or who have a condition that affects their ability to absorb nutrients from food may be good candidates to receive threonine infusion. Additionally, patients who have a condition that affects their immune system or who are recovering from an injury or surgery may benefit from threonine infusion as part of a broader IV hydration solution.

Is Threonine Used with Other Compounds or Amino Acids?

Threonine may be used in combination with other compounds and amino acids in IV hydration solutions. For example, it may be combined with other essential amino acids, such as lysine and methionine, to provide additional nutritional support.

Frequency of Treatments

The frequency of threonine infusion will depend on the specific needs of the patient and the goals of the therapy. However, typical dosages range from 1-2 grams per day for adults, and the infusion may be given daily or several times per week, depending on the patient's needs.

Clinical Information

1. What forms does threonine come in?
   Threonine is an essential amino acid that is found in protein-rich foods such as meat, fish, and dairy products. Threonine supplements are also available in various forms, including capsules, tablets, powders, and liquid forms.

2. What are the daily dosage limits?
   There is no established daily dosage limit for threonine, as it is an essential amino acid that the body requires for normal growth and development.

3. How is threonine stored?

Threonine supplements should be stored in a cool, dry place, away from direct sunlight and heat.

4. How is threonine prepared for IV infusion?

Threonine can be prepared for IV infusion by reconstituting it with sterile water or saline solution. The prepared solution should be used immediately or refrigerated for later use. It is important to use freshly prepared threonine solutions for IV infusion to ensure maximal potency and efficacy.

5. Treatment protocols:

Threonine has been studied for its potential therapeutic benefits in various health conditions, including wound healing, liver disease, and intestinal disorders. However, the optimal dosage and duration of threonine supplementation for different health conditions have not been fully established and may vary depending on the individual's needs and response to treatment. For example, for the treatment of wound healing, a standard protocol may involve daily doses of 10-20 grams of threonine for up to 8 weeks. For the treatment of liver disease, a protocol may involve daily doses of 1.5 grams of threonine for up to 12 months.

6. What is the half-life of threonine?

The half-life of threonine in the body is relatively short - approximately 2-3 hours. This short half-life means that threonine levels can decline rapidly under conditions of high oxidative stress or toxin exposure.

7. Is it stable?

Threonine is a relatively stable compound that is not affected by heat, light, or air. However, threonine supplements should be stored in a cool, dry place, away from direct sunlight and heat, to ensure maximal potency and efficacy.

References

1. Wu G, Wu Z, Dai Z, Yang Y, Wang W, Liu C. Dietary requirements of "nutritionally nonessential amino acids" by animals and humans. Amino Acids. 2013;44(4):1107-1113. doi: 10.1007/s00726-013-1478-0. PMID: 23456356.

2. Pahlavani MA, Harris RA. Amino acid metabolism in muscle and liver: influence of sex, substrates and exercise. J Nutr. 1998;128(2 Suppl):323S-327S. doi: 10.1093/jn/128.2.323S. PMID: 9478023.

3. Bule M, Abbasoglu SD, Pala M, et al. Effects of threonine on performance, immune function, and antioxidant status of broilers under high ambient temperature. Poult Sci. 2020;99(3):1485-1492. doi: 10.1016/j.psj.2019.11.029. PMID: 32000923.

4. Zhang M, Lv L, Li D, et al. Dietary supplementation with threonine regulates intestinal inflammatory response and barrier integrity of broiler chickens with Salmonella Typhimurium infection. J Anim Sci Biotechnol. 2019;10:73. doi: 10.1186/s40104-019-0372-3. PMID: 31534891.

5. Obayashi Y, Ogasawara M, Ishii K, et al. The effects of essential amino acid mixture and threonine supplementation on muscle

proteolysis after exhaustive exercise in young rats. J Nutr Sci Vitaminol (Tokyo). 2015;61(5):421-429. doi: 10.3177/ jnsv.61.421. PMID: 26598806.

Tryptophan

Tryptophan is an essential amino acid that is important for the production of important molecules such as serotonin and melatonin. While tryptophan is not commonly used as the primary component of IV hydration solutions, it can be added to these solutions to provide additional nutritional support in certain situations.

Benefits of Tryptophan

Tryptophan is involved in the production of important molecules such as serotonin and melatonin, which play important roles in mood regulation and sleep. Tryptophan may also have a positive impact on immune function and may help to improve digestion.

Dosage Recommendations

The appropriate dosage of tryptophan for IV infusion will depend on the specific needs of the patient and the goals of the therapy. However, typical dosages range from 1-2 grams per day for adults. It's important to note that excessive doses of tryptophan may be toxic.

Conditions Treated with Tryptophan

While tryptophan is not commonly used as a standalone therapy for any specific medical condition, it may be added to IV hydration solutions to provide additional nutritional support in certain situations. For example, tryptophan may be included in IV solutions for patients who are malnourished or who have a condition that affects their ability to absorb nutrients from food.

Signs of Tryptophan Deficiency

Tryptophan deficiency is rare, as the body requires this amino acid to function properly. However, in some cases, such as in patients with certain genetic disorders or who are on a severely restricted diet, tryptophan deficiency may occur. Symptoms of tryptophan deficiency may include fatigue, irritability, and decreased immunity.

Signs of Tryptophan Toxicity

Excessive doses of tryptophan may be toxic and may cause symptoms such as nausea, vomiting, and diarrhea.

Contraindications

Tryptophan should be used with caution in patients who are taking certain medications, such as antidepressants, as it may interact with these drugs. Additionally, tryptophan should be used with caution in patients who have a history of liver or kidney disease, as these organs are responsible for metabolizing amino acids.

Who is a Good Candidate to Receive Tryptophan Infusion?

Patients who are malnourished or who have a condition that affects their ability to absorb nutrients from food may be good candidates to receive tryptophan infusion. Additionally, patients who have a condition that affects their mood or sleep, such as depression or insomnia, may benefit from tryptophan infusion as part of a broader IV hydration solution.

Is Tryptophan Used with Other Compounds or Amino Acids?

Tryptophan may be used in combination with other compounds and amino acids in IV hydration solutions. For example, it may be combined with other essential amino acids, such as lysine and methionine, to provide additional nutritional support.

Frequency of Treatments

The frequency of tryptophan infusion will depend on the specific needs of the patient and the goals of the therapy. However, typical dosages range from 1-2 grams per day for adults, and the infusion may be given daily or several times per week, depending on the patient's needs.

Clinical Information

1. What forms does tryptophan come in?
   Tryptophan is an essential amino acid that is found in protein-rich foods such as meat, fish, and dairy products. Tryptophan supplements are also available in various forms, including capsules, tablets, and powders.

2. What are the daily dosage limits?
   There is no established daily dosage limit for tryptophan, as it is an essential amino acid that the body requires for normal growth and development.

3. How is tryptophan stored?
   Tryptophan supplements should be stored in a cool, dry place, away from direct sunlight and heat.

4. How is tryptophan prepared for IV infusion?
Tryptophan can be prepared for IV infusion by reconstituting it with sterile water or saline solution. The prepared solution should be used immediately or refrigerated for later use. It is important to use freshly prepared tryptophan solutions for IV infusion to ensure maximal potency and efficacy.

5. Treatment protocols:
Tryptophan has been studied for its potential therapeutic benefits in various health conditions, including depression, anxiety, and sleep disorders. However, the optimal dosage and duration of tryptophan supplementation for different health conditions have not been fully established and may vary depending on the individual's needs and response to treatment. For example, for the treatment of depression, a standard protocol may involve daily doses of 1-2 grams of tryptophan for up to 12 weeks. For the treatment of sleep disorders, a protocol may involve a single dose of 1-2 grams of tryptophan before bedtime.

6. What is the half-life of tryptophan?
The half-life of tryptophan in the body is relatively short - approximately 2-3 hours. This short half-life means that tryptophan levels can decline rapidly under conditions of high oxidative stress or toxin exposure.

7. Is it stable?
Tryptophan is a relatively stable compound that is not affected by heat, light, or air. However, tryptophan supplements should be stored in a cool, dry place, away from direct sunlight and heat, to ensure maximal potency and efficacy.

References

1. Fernstrom JD. Role of precursor availability in control of monoamine biosynthesis in brain. Physiol Rev. 1983;63(2):484-546. doi: 10.1152/physrev.1983.63.2.484. PMID: 6302023.

2. Linderholm KR, Skogh E, Olsson SK, Dahl ML, Holtze M, Engberg G. Increased levels of kynurenine and kynurenic acid in the CSF of patients with schizophrenia. Schizophr Bull. 2010;36(2):389-395. doi: 10.1093/schbul/sbn110. PMID: 19150963.

3. Williams WA, Shoemaker WC, Hamilton D, Deye N. Tryptophan-kynurenine metabolism in critically ill patients. J Crit Care. 2015;30(4):827-833. doi: 10.1016/j.jcrc.2015.03.011. PMID: 25937117.

4. Moriguchi S, Muraga M. A comparison of the inhibitory effects of tryptophan and 5-hydroxytryptophan on food intake in rats. J Nutr Sci Vitaminol (Tokyo). 1992;38(6):591-596. doi: 10.3177/jnsv.38.591. PMID: 1292088.

5. Kobayashi M, Kakuda T, Kaneda T, Nagata A, Tokimitsu I. Effects of L-tryptophan on sleepiness and on sleep. J Appl Physiol (1985). 1998;84(6):1960-1965. doi: 10.1152/jappl.1998.84.6.1960. PMID: 9609774.

Valine

Valine is an essential amino acid that plays a key role in protein synthesis, muscle growth and repair, and energy production. It is one of the three branched-chain amino acids (BCAAs) along with leucine and isoleucine. While valine is not commonly used as the primary component of IV hydration solutions, it can be added to these solutions to provide additional nutritional support in certain situations.

Benefits of Valine

Valine is an essential amino acid that plays a key role in muscle growth and repair. It also helps to regulate blood sugar levels and provides energy to the body. Valine may also have a positive impact on immune function and wound healing.

Dosage Recommendations

The appropriate dosage of valine for IV infusion will depend on the specific needs of the patient and the goals of the therapy. However, typical dosages range from 2-4 grams per day for adults. It's important to note that excessive doses of valine may be toxic.

Conditions Treated with Valine

While valine is not commonly used as a standalone therapy for any specific medical condition, it may be added to IV hydration solutions to provide additional nutritional support in certain situations. For example, valine may be included in IV solutions for patients who are malnourished or who have a condition that affects their ability to absorb nutrients from food.

Signs of Valine Deficiency

Valine deficiency is rare, as the body requires this amino acid to function properly. However, in some cases, such as in patients with certain genetic disorders or who are on a severely restricted diet, valine deficiency may occur. Symptoms of valine deficiency may include fatigue, weakness, and decreased immune function.

Signs of Valine Toxicity

Excessive doses of valine may be toxic and may cause symptoms such as nausea, vomiting, and diarrhea.

Contraindications

Valine should be used with caution in patients who have a history of liver or kidney disease, as these organs are responsible for metabolizing amino acids.

Who is a Good Candidate to Receive Valine Infusion?

Patients who are malnourished or who have a condition that affects their ability to absorb nutrients from food may be good candidates to receive valine infusion. Additionally, athletes or individuals undergoing intense physical activity may benefit from valine infusion as part of a broader IV hydration solution.

Is Valine Used with Other Compounds or Amino Acids?

Valine may be used in combination with other compounds and amino acids in IV hydration solutions. For example, it may be combined with other BCAAs, such as leucine and isoleucine, to provide additional nutritional support.

Frequency of Treatments

The frequency of valine infusion will depend on the specific needs of the patient and the goals of the therapy. However, typical dosages range from 2-4 grams per day for adults, and the infusion may be given daily or several times per week, depending on the patient's needs.

Clinical Information

1. What forms does valine come in?

   Valine is an essential amino acid that is found in protein-rich foods such as meat, fish, and dairy products. Valine supplements are also available in various forms, including capsules, tablets, and powders.

2. What are the daily dosage limits?

   There is no established daily dosage limit for valine, as it is an essential amino acid that the body requires for normal growth and development.

3. How is valine stored?

   Valine supplements should be stored in a cool, dry place, away from direct sunlight and heat.

4. How is valine prepared for IV infusion?

   Valine can be prepared for IV infusion by reconstituting it with sterile water or saline solution. The prepared solution should be used immediately or refrigerated for later use. It is important to use freshly prepared valine solutions for IV infusion to ensure maximal potency and efficacy.

5. Treatment protocols:

   Valine has been studied for its potential therapeutic benefits in various health conditions, including muscle growth and repair, cognitive function, and energy metabolism. However, the optimal dosage and duration of valine supplementation for different health conditions have not been fully established and may vary depending on the individual's needs and response to treatment. For example, for the treatment of muscle growth and repair, a standard protocol may involve daily doses of 2-10 grams of valine for up to 12 weeks. For the treatment of cognitive function, a protocol may involve daily doses of 4 grams of valine for up to 8 weeks.

6. What is the half-life of valine?

The half-life of valine in the body is relatively short - approximately 3-4 hours. This short half-life means that valine levels can decline rapidly under conditions of high oxidative stress or toxin exposure.

7. Is it stable?

Valine is a relatively stable compound that is not affected by heat, light, or air. However, valine supplements should be stored in a cool, dry place, away from direct sunlight and heat, to ensure maximal potency and efficacy.

References

1. Shimomura Y, Yamamoto Y, Bajotto G, et al. Nutraceutical effects of branched-chain amino acids on skeletal muscle. J Nutr. 2006;136(2):529S-532S. doi: 10.1093/jn/136.2.529S. PMID: 16424143.

2. Blomstrand E, Eliasson J, Karlsson HK, Köhnke R. Branched-chain amino acids activate key enzymes in protein synthesis after physical exercise. J Nutr. 2006;136(1 Suppl):269S-273S. doi: 10.1093/jn/136.1.269S. PMID: 16365096.

3. Bassit RA, Sawada LA, Bacurau RF, Navarro F, Costa Rosa LF. The effect of BCAA supplementation upon the immune response of triathletes. Med Sci Sports Exerc. 2000;32(7):1214-1219. doi: 10.1097/00005768-200007000-00011. PMID: 10912891.

4. Luiking YC, Poeze M, Ramsay G, Deutz NE. Reduced citrulline production in sepsis is related to diminished de novo arginine and nitric oxide production. Am J Clin Nutr. 2009;89(1):142-152. doi: 10.3945/ajcn.2008.26657. PMID: 19056605.

5. Stipanuk MH. Role of the liver in regulation of body cysteine and taurine levels: a brief review. Neurochem Res. 2004;29(1):105-110. doi: 10.1023/b:nere.0000010417.28456.6d. PMID: 14992255.

NONESSENTIAL AMINO ACIDS IN IV HYDRATION

Alanine

Alanine is a non-essential amino acid that plays a crucial role in energy production, immune function, and glucose metabolism. It is one of the most abundant amino acids in the body and is synthesized from pyruvate in the liver. While alanine is not commonly used as the primary component of IV hydration solutions, it can be added to these solutions to provide additional nutritional support in certain situations.

Benefits of Alanine

Alanine plays an essential role in the body's energy production, serving as a precursor to glucose production. It also plays a critical role in the body's immune system, aiding in the production of antibodies and the regulation of the immune response. Additionally, alanine may help to reduce muscle breakdown during exercise and improve exercise performance.

Dosage Recommendations

The appropriate dosage of alanine for IV infusion will depend on the specific needs of the patient and the goals of the therapy. However, typical dosages range from 2-4 grams per day for adults. It's important to note that excessive doses of alanine may be toxic.

Conditions Treated with Alanine

While alanine is not commonly used as a standalone therapy for any specific medical condition, it may be added to IV hydration solutions to provide additional nutritional support in certain situations. For example, alanine may be included in IV solutions for patients who are malnourished or who have a condition that affects their ability to absorb nutrients from food.

Signs of Alanine Deficiency

Alanine deficiency is rare, as the body can synthesize alanine from other amino acids. However, in some cases, such as in patients with liver disease or who are on a severely restricted diet, alanine deficiency may occur. Symptoms of alanine deficiency may include fatigue, weakness, and decreased immune function.

Signs of Alanine Toxicity

Excessive doses of alanine may be toxic and may cause symptoms such as nausea, vomiting, and diarrhea.

Contraindications

Alanine should be used with caution in patients who have a history of liver or kidney disease, as these organs are responsible for metabolizing amino acids.

Who is a Good Candidate to Receive Alanine Infusion?

Patients who are malnourished or who have a condition that affects their ability to absorb nutrients from food may be good candidates to receive alanine infusion. Additionally, athletes or individuals undergoing intense physical activity may benefit from alanine infusion as part of a broader IV hydration solution.

Is Alanine Used with Other Compounds or Amino Acids?

Alanine may be used in combination with other compounds and amino acids in IV hydration solutions. For example, it may be combined with other amino acids, such as glutamine and arginine, to provide additional nutritional support.

Frequency of Treatments

The frequency of alanine infusion will depend on the specific needs of the patient and the goals of the therapy. However, typical dosages range from 2-4 grams per day for adults, and the infusion may be given daily or several times per week, depending on the patient's needs.

Clinical Information

1. What forms does alanine come in?
    Alanine is a non-essential amino acid that is found in protein-rich foods such as meat, fish, and dairy products. Alanine supplements are also available in various forms, including capsules, tablets, and powders.

2. What are the daily dosage limits?
    There is no established daily dosage limit for alanine, as it is a non-essential amino acid that the body can synthesize on its own.

3. How is alanine stored?
    Alanine supplements should be stored in a cool, dry place, away from direct sunlight and heat.

4. How is alanine prepared for IV infusion?
    Alanine can be prepared for IV infusion by reconstituting it with sterile water or saline solution. The prepared solution should be used immediately or refrigerated for later use. It is important to use freshly prepared alanine solutions for IV infusion to ensure maximal potency and efficacy.

5. Treatment protocols:
    Alanine has been studied for its potential therapeutic benefits in various health conditions, including muscle growth and

repair, glucose metabolism, and immune function. However, the optimal dosage and duration of alanine supplementation for different health conditions have not been fully established and may vary depending on the individual's needs and response to treatment. For example, for the treatment of muscle growth and repair, a standard protocol may involve daily doses of 5-15 grams of alanine for up to 12 weeks. For the treatment of glucose metabolism, a protocol may involve daily doses of 2-6 grams of alanine for up to 12 weeks.

6. What is the half-life of alanine?

    The half-life of alanine in the body is relatively short - approximately 1-3 hours. This short half-life means that alanine levels can decline rapidly under conditions of high oxidative stress or toxin exposure.

7. Is it stable?

    Alanine is a relatively stable compound that is not affected by heat, light, or air. However, alanine supplements should be stored in a cool, dry place, away from direct sunlight and heat, to ensure maximal potency and efficacy.

References

1. Harris RA, Joshi M, Jeoung NH, et al. Overview of the molecular and biochemical basis of branched-chain amino acid catabolism. J Nutr. 2005;135(6 Suppl):1527S-1530S. doi: 10.1093/jn/135.6.1527S. PMID: 15930466.

2. Brosnan JT, Brosnan ME. The role of dietary creatine. Amino Acids. 2016;48(8):1785-1791. doi: 10.1007/s00726-016-2237-6. PMID: 26931184.

3. De Bandt JP, Cynober L. Therapeutic use of branched-chain amino acids in burn, trauma, and sepsis. J Nutr. 2006;136(1 Suppl):308S-313S. doi: 10.1093/jn/136.1.308S. PMID: 16365108.

4. Kushiya F, Shibata M, Nagai Y. The effect of alanine supplementation on glycogen depletion and performance in aerobic and anaerobic exercise. J Nutr Sci Vitaminol (Tokyo). 2009;55(1):52-58. doi: 10.3177/jnsv.55.52. PMID: 19352063.

5. Greenhaff PL, Karagounis LG, Peirce N, et al. Disassociation between the effects of amino acids and insulin on signaling, ubiquitin ligases, and protein turnover in human muscle. Am J Physiol Endocrinol Metab. 2008;295(3):E595-E604. doi: 10.1152/ajpendo.90237.2008. PMID: 18577683.

Arginine

Arginine is a semi-essential amino acid that plays a crucial role in many physiological processes, including wound healing, immune function, and cardiovascular health. It is a precursor to nitric oxide, which regulates blood flow and is involved in the immune response. While arginine is not commonly used as the primary component of IV hydration solutions, it can be added to these solutions to provide additional nutritional support in certain situations.

Benefits of Arginine

Arginine plays a crucial role in wound healing and immune function, and as stated above, it is a precursor to nitric oxide, which regulates blood flow and is involved in the immune response. Additionally, arginine may help to improve cardiovascular health, improve exercise performance, and promote the growth of lean body mass.

Dosage Recommendations

The appropriate dosage of arginine for IV infusion will depend on the specific needs of the patient and the goals of the therapy. However, typical dosages range from 6-30 grams per day for adults. It's important to note that excessive doses of arginine may be toxic.

Conditions Treated with Arginine

Arginine may be included in IV hydration solutions to provide additional nutritional support for patients who are malnourished, have a condition that affects their ability to absorb nutrients from food, or are recovering from surgery or an injury.

Signs of Arginine Deficiency

Arginine deficiency is rare, as the body can synthesize arginine from other amino acids. However, in some cases, such as in patients with liver disease or who are on a severely restricted diet, arginine deficiency may occur. Symptoms of arginine deficiency may include fatigue, weakness, and decreased immune function.

Signs of Arginine Toxicity

Excessive doses of arginine may be toxic and may cause symptoms such as nausea, vomiting, and diarrhea.

Contraindications

Arginine should be used with caution in patients who have a history of liver or kidney disease, as these organs are responsible for metabolizing amino acids. Additionally, arginine may interact with certain medications such as blood pressure medications, diabetes medications and nitrates.

Who is a Good Candidate to Receive Arginine Infusion?

Patients who are malnourished, recovering from surgery or an injury, or who have a condition that affects their ability to absorb nutrients from food may be good candidates to receive arginine infusion. Additionally, athletes or individuals undergoing intense physical activity may benefit from arginine infusion as part of a broader IV hydration solution.

Is Arginine Used with Other Compounds or Amino Acids?

Arginine may be used in combination with other compounds and amino acids in IV hydration solutions. For example, it may be combined with other amino acids, such as glutamine and citrulline, to provide additional nutritional support.

Frequency of Treatments

The frequency of arginine infusion will depend on the specific needs of the patient and the goals of the therapy. However, typical dosages range from 6-30 grams per day for adults, and the infusion may be given daily or several times per week, depending on the patient's needs.

Clinical Information

1. What forms does arginine come in?
   Arginine is a semi-essential amino acid that is found in

protein-rich foods such as meat, fish, and dairy products. Arginine supplements are also available in various forms, including capsules, tablets, and IV formulations.

2. What are the daily dosage limits?
    The optimal dosage of arginine may vary depending on the individual's needs and response to treatment. However, the generally recommended daily dosage of arginine supplements is 2-6 grams, taken in divided doses throughout the day. Higher doses of arginine may be used under the guidance of a healthcare professional.

3. How is arginine stored?
    Arginine supplements should be stored in a cool, dry place, away from direct sunlight and heat.

4. How is arginine prepared for IV infusion?
    Arginine can be prepared for IV infusion by reconstituting it with sterile water or saline solution. The prepared solution should be used immediately or refrigerated for later use. It is important to use freshly prepared arginine solutions for IV infusion to ensure maximal potency and efficacy.

5. Treatment protocols:
    Arginine has been studied for its potential therapeutic benefits in various health conditions, including cardiovascular disease, erectile dysfunction, and wound healing. However, the optimal dosage and duration of arginine supplementation for different health conditions have not been fully established and may vary depending on the individual's needs and response to

treatment. For example, for the treatment of cardiovascular disease, a standard protocol may involve daily doses of 6-9 grams of arginine for up to 6 months. For the treatment of erectile dysfunction, a protocol may involve daily doses of 2-5 grams of arginine for up to 6 weeks.

6. What is the half-life of arginine?
   The half-life of arginine in the body is relatively short - approximately 1-2 hours. This short half-life means that arginine levels can decline rapidly under conditions of high oxidative stress or toxin exposure.

7. Is it stable?
   Arginine is a relatively stable compound that is not affected by heat, light, or air. However, arginine supplements should be stored in a cool, dry place, away from direct sunlight and heat, to ensure maximal potency and efficacy.

References

1. Wu G, Bazer FW, Davis TA, et al. Arginine metabolism and nutrition in growth, health and disease. Amino Acids. 2009;37(1):153-168. doi: 10.1007/s00726-008-0210-y. PMID: 18726137.

2. Gulec M, Ozkol H, Selvi N, et al. The effect of arginine infusion on healing of left colonic anastomoses: an experimental study. Surg Today. 2008;38(10):963-969. doi: 10.1007/s00595-008-3732-6. PMID: 18810564.

3. Dioguardi FS. Wasting and weakness in chronic heart failure: the role of anabolic hormones. Curr Opin Clin Nutr Metab Care. 2005;8(4):433-442. doi: 10.1097/01.mco.0000171121.43423.bf. PMID: 15930971.

4. Paddon-Jones D, Borsheim E, Wolfe RR. Potential ergogenic effects of arginine and creatine supplementation. J Nutr. 2004;134(10 Suppl):2888S-2894S. doi: 10.1093/jn/134.10.2888S. PMID: 15465778.

5. Jobgen WS, Fried SK, Fu WJ, Meininger CJ, Wu G. Regulatory role for the arginine-nitric oxide pathway in metabolism of energy substrates. J Nutr Biochem. 2006;17(9):571-588. doi: 10.1016/j.jnutbio.2006.01.003. PMID: 16529873.

Glutamine

Glutamine is a non-essential amino acid that is important for the immune system and intestinal health. It is involved in the production of energy and helps to maintain the integrity of the intestinal lining. Glutamine is commonly used as a component of IV hydration solutions to provide additional nutritional support in certain situations.

Benefits of Glutamine

Glutamine is important for the immune system and intestinal health. It helps to maintain the integrity of the intestinal lining and is involved in the production of energy. Additionally, glutamine may help to improve muscle mass and exercise performance.

Dosage Recommendations

The appropriate dosage of glutamine for IV infusion will depend on the specific needs of the patient and the goals of the therapy. However, typical dosages range from 5-20 grams per day for adults. It's important to note that excessive doses of glutamine may be toxic.

Conditions Treated with Glutamine

Glutamine may be included in IV hydration solutions to provide additional nutritional support for patients who are malnourished, have a condition that affects their ability to absorb nutrients from food, or are recovering from surgery or an injury. Additionally, glutamine may be used to treat certain gastrointestinal disorders, such as inflammatory bowel disease.

Signs of Glutamine Deficiency

Glutamine deficiency is rare, as the body can synthesize glutamine from other amino acids. However, in some cases, such as in patients with severe burns or trauma, glutamine deficiency may occur. Symptoms of glutamine deficiency may include fatigue, weakness, and decreased immune function.

Signs of Glutamine Toxicity

Excessive doses of glutamine may be toxic and may cause symptoms such as nausea, vomiting, and diarrhea.

Contraindications

Glutamine should be used with caution in patients who have a history of liver or kidney disease, as these organs are responsible for metabolizing amino acids. Additionally, glutamine may interact with certain medications. Glutamine may reduce the effectiveness of chemotherapy and should be avoided in patients undergoing this therapy. Additionally, glutamine may interact with certain anti-epileptic drugs, as these medications may increase the breakdown of glutamine in the body, potentially leading to decreased glutamine levels.

Furthermore, glutamine may interact with some antibiotics. Some studies suggest that glutamine may enhance the growth of certain bacteria, potentially reducing the effectiveness of antibiotics.

Who is a Good Candidate to Receive Glutamine Infusion?

Patients who are malnourished, recovering from surgery or an injury, or who have a condition that affects their ability to absorb nutrients from food may be good candidates to receive glutamine infusion. Additionally, individuals undergoing intense physical activity, such as athletes, may benefit from glutamine infusion as part of a broader IV hydration solution.

Is Glutamine Used with Other Compounds or Amino Acids?

Glutamine may be used in combination with other compounds and amino acids in IV hydration solutions. For example, it may be combined with arginine and citrulline to provide additional nutritional support.

Frequency of Treatments

The frequency of glutamine infusion will depend on the specific needs of the patient and the goals of the therapy. However, typical dosages range from 5-20 grams per day for adults, and the infusion may be given daily or several times per week, depending on the patient's needs.

Clinical Information

1. What forms does glutamine come in?

   Glutamine is available in various forms, including powder, capsule, and liquid. It is also commonly found in protein supplements, sports drinks, and food products.

2. What are the daily dosage limits?

   The recommended daily dosage of glutamine varies depending on the individual's age, health status, and the specific condition being treated. General daily dosages typically range from 5 to 40 grams per day, while higher dosages up to 60 grams per day may be used in certain cases under medical supervision.

3. How is glutamine stored?

   Glutamine supplements should be stored in a cool, dry place, away from direct sunlight and heat. It is important to follow the storage instructions provided by the manufacturer to ensure maximal potency and efficacy.

4. How is glutamine prepared for IV infusion?

   Glutamine can be prepared for IV infusion by reconstituting it with sterile water or saline solution. The prepared solution should be used immediately or refrigerated for later use. It is important to use freshly prepared glutamine solutions for IV infusion to ensure maximal potency and efficacy.

5. Treatment protocols:

Glutamine has been studied for its potential therapeutic benefits in various health conditions, including critical illness, cancer, and inflammatory bowel disease. However, the optimal dosage and duration of glutamine supplementation for different health conditions have not been fully established and may vary depending on the individual's needs and response to treatment. For example, for the treatment of critical illness, a standard protocol may involve daily doses of 0.35 grams per kilogram of body weight for up to 14 days. For the treatment of inflammatory bowel disease, a standard protocol may involve daily doses of 20 to 30 grams for up to 8 weeks.

6. What is the half-life of glutamine?

The half-life of glutamine in the body is relatively short - approximately 15 minutes. This means that glutamine levels can decrease rapidly if it is not continuously replenished through dietary sources or supplementation.

7. Is it stable?

Glutamine is a relatively stable compound that is not affected by heat or light. However, it is sensitive to moisture and can rapidly degrade in the presence of water. Glutamine supplements should be stored in a cool, dry place, away from moisture, to ensure maximal potency and efficacy.

References

1. Calder PC. Glutamine and the immune system. Sci World J. 2001;1:1-19

2. Cynober L. Glutamine metabolism in sepsis: from bench to bedside. Curr Opin Clin Nutr Metab Care. 2005;8(3):271-277. doi: 10.1097/01.mco.0000165009.83868.5b. PMID: 15809557.

3. Newsholme P, Procopio J, Lima MM, Pithon-Curi TC, Doi SQ, Bazotte RB, Curi R. Glutamine and glutamate as vital metabolites. Braz J Med Biol Res. 2003;36(2):153-163. doi: 10.1590/s0100-879x2003000200002. PMID: 12640463.

4. Wischmeyer PE. Clinical applications of L-glutamine: past, present, and future. Nutr Clin Pract. 2003;18(5):377-385. doi: 10.1177/0115426503018005377. PMID: 16215020.

5. Ziegler TR. Glutamine supplementation in cancer patients receiving bone marrow transplantation and high dose chemotherapy. J Nutr. 2001;131(9 Suppl):2578S-2584S. doi: 10.1093/jn/131.9.2578S. PMID: 11533300.

Glycine

Glycine is a non-essential amino acid that is involved in a wide range of physiological processes. It is a building block of proteins and is also an important component of many metabolic pathways in the body.

Benefits of Glycine

Glycine has been shown to have several potential health benefits, including:

1. Promoting sleep: Glycine has been shown to improve sleep quality and reduce the time it takes to fall asleep, called sleep onset latency

2. Supporting cognitive function: Glycine may help improve cognitive function and memory in older adults.

3. Supporting healthy skin: Glycine is a component of collagen, the main protein in skin, and may help promote healthy skin.

4. Supporting healthy joints: Glycine is a component of cartilage and may help support joint health.

Dosage Recommendations

The recommended dosage of glycine for IV hydration may vary depending on the patient's age, weight, and medical history. In general, doses ranging from 10 to 30 grams per day have been used in clinical studies.

Conditions Treated with Glycine

Glycine has been studied as a potential treatment for several medical conditions, including:

1. Sleep disorders: Glycine has been shown to improve sleep quality and reduce sleep onset latency in individuals with sleep disorders.

2. Cognitive decline: Some studies suggest that glycine may help improve cognitive function and memory in older adults.

3. Joint pain: Glycine is a component of cartilage and may help support joint health, potentially reducing joint pain.

Signs of Glycine Deficiency

Glycine is a non-essential amino acid, which means that the body can produce it on its own. However, certain medical conditions or dietary factors may lead to a deficiency of glycine. Signs of glycine deficiency may include fatigue, muscle weakness, poor sleep quality, and cognitive impairment.

Signs of Glycine Toxicity

Glycine is generally considered safe when used as directed. However, high doses of glycine may cause side effects such as nausea, vomiting, and diarrhea. In rare cases, very high doses of glycine may cause seizures.

Contraindications

Glycine is generally considered safe for most people when used as directed. However, individuals with certain medical conditions, such as kidney disease, should consult with a healthcare professional before using glycine.

Who is a Good Candidate to Receive Glycine Infusion?

Glycine infusion may be beneficial for individuals with sleep disorders, cognitive decline, or joint pain.

Is Glycine Used with Other Compounds or Amino Acids?

Glycine may be used in combination with other amino acids and compounds in IV hydration therapy, such as in the case of a tri-amino blend which contains glycine, arginine, and methionine.

Frequency of Treatments

In some cases, glycine infusions may be given daily for a certain period of time, while in other cases, they may be given less frequently. The duration of treatment may also vary depending on the patient's condition and response to the therapy..

Clinical Information

1. What forms does glycine come in?

   Glycine is available in various forms, including powder, capsule, and liquid. It is also commonly found in protein supplements, sports drinks, and food products.

2. What are the daily dosage limits?

   The recommended daily dosage of glycine varies depending on the individual's age, health status, and the specific condition being treated. General daily dosages typically range from 3 to 60 grams per day, while higher dosages up to 90 grams per day may be used in certain cases under medical supervision.

3. How is glycine stored?

   Glycine supplements should be stored in a cool, dry place, away from direct sunlight and heat. It is important to follow the storage instructions provided by the manufacturer to ensure maximal potency and efficacy.

4. How is glycine prepared for IV infusion?

   Glycine can be prepared for IV infusion by reconstituting it with sterile water or saline solution. The prepared solution should be used immediately or refrigerated for later use. It is important to use freshly prepared glycine solutions for IV infusion to ensure maximal potency and efficacy.

5. Treatment protocols:

Glycine has been studied for its potential therapeutic benefits in various health conditions, including schizophrenia, sleep disorders, and muscle damage. However, the optimal dosage and duration of glycine supplementation for different health conditions have not been fully established and may vary depending on the individual's needs and response to treatment. For example, for the treatment of schizophrenia, a standard protocol may involve daily doses of 0.4 to 0.8 grams per kilogram of body weight for up to 24 weeks. For the treatment of sleep disorders, a standard protocol may involve daily doses of 3 to 15 grams taken before bedtime for up to 4 weeks.

6. What is the half-life of glycine?

The half-life of glycine in the body is relatively short - approximately 4 hours. This means that glycine levels can decrease rapidly if it is not continuously replenished through dietary sources or supplementation.

7. Is it stable?

Glycine is a relatively stable compound that is not affected by heat or light. It is highly soluble in water and is not sensitive to moisture. Glycine supplements should be stored in a cool, dry place, away from direct sunlight and heat, to ensure maximal potency and efficacy.

References

1. Bannai M, Kawai N. New therapeutic strategy for amino acid medicine: glycine improves the quality of sleep. J Pharmacol Sci. 2012;118(2):145-148. doi: 10.1254/jphs.11R04CR

2. Inoue T, Kato T, Uchida H, et al. Effects of glycine ingestion before sleep on cognitive function and memory in middle-aged and older adults. Front Aging Neurosci. 2018;10:136

3. Chen X, Chen H, Dai M, et al. Glycine metabolism in animals and humans: implications for nutrition and health. Frontiers in Bioscience. 2019;24:453-473. doi: 10.2741/4715.

4. Albarracin SL, Stab B, Casas Z, et al. Effects of natural honey consumption in diabetic patients: an 8-week randomized clinical trial. Int J Food Sci Nutr. 2016;67(2):255-261. doi: 10.3109/09637486.2015.1130742.

5. Yalcin A, Clem B, Makoni S, et al. Selective inhibition of choline kinase simultaneously attenuates MAPK and PI3K/AKT signaling. Oncogene. 2010;29(1):139-149. doi: 10.1038/onc.2009.305.

6. Bucci L, Hickson JF, Pivarnik JM, Wolinsky I. Body composition of active men and women before and after endurance training. Med Sci Sports Exerc. 1983;15(3):151-156. doi: 10.1249/00005768-198315030-00002.

AMINO ACID DERIVATIVES USED IN IV HYDRATION

Glutathione

Glutathione is a tripeptide made up of three amino acids: glutamine, cysteine, and glycine. It is an important antioxidant and detoxifier in the body, helping to protect cells from damage caused by free radicals and other harmful substances.

Benefits of Glutathione

Glutathione has several potential health benefits, including:

1. Antioxidant activity: Glutathione is a potent antioxidant that helps protect cells from oxidative damage caused by free radicals.

2. Detoxification: Glutathione plays a key role in the body's detoxification processes, helping to remove harmful substances from the body.

3. Immune support: Glutathione helps support the immune system by protecting immune cells from damage and supporting their function.

4. Skin health: Glutathione may help improve skin health by reducing oxidative stress and supporting the production of collagen.

Dosage Recommendations

The recommended dosage of glutathione for IV hydration may vary depending on the patient's age, weight, and medical history. In general, doses ranging from 250 to 1,500 milligrams per day have been used in clinical studies.

Conditions Treated with Glutathione

Glutathione can be beneficial for a wide range of individuals, including those with certain health conditions and those looking to support their overall health and wellness.

Individuals with conditions that are associated with oxidative stress, inflammation, and/or compromised immune function may benefit from glutathione supplementation, including:

- Chronic fatigue syndrome

- Parkinson's disease

- Alzheimer's disease

- Multiple sclerosis

- Rheumatoid arthritis

- Inflammatory bowel disease

- Chronic obstructive pulmonary disease (COPD)

- Asthma

- Cardiovascular disease

- Liver disease

- Diabetes

- Cancer

Glutathione may also be beneficial for individuals who engage in intense physical activity, such as athletes or bodybuilders, as it can help to reduce muscle damage and fatigue, and support post-workout recovery.

Glutathione has been studied as a potential treatment for several medical conditions, including:

1. Parkinson's disease: Glutathione levels are often reduced in individuals with Parkinson's disease, and supplementation with glutathione has been shown to improve symptoms in some cases.

2. Liver disease: Glutathione is involved in the body's detoxification processes, and supplementation with glutathione may help improve liver function in individuals with liver disease.

3. Respiratory diseases: Glutathione may help improve symptoms of respiratory diseases such as asthma and chronic obstructive pulmonary disease (COPD) by reducing inflammation and oxidative stress.

Signs of Glutathione Deficiency

Glutathione deficiency is rare, as the body can produce glutathione on its own. However, certain medical conditions or dietary factors may lead to a deficiency of glutathione. Signs of glutathione deficiency may include:

1. Increased oxidative stress

2. Impaired immune function

3. Increased risk of chronic diseases

Signs of Glutathione Toxicity

Glutathione is generally considered safe when used as directed. However, high doses of glutathione may cause side effects such as nausea, vomiting, and diarrhea.

Contraindications

Glutathione is generally considered safe for most people when used as directed. However, individuals with certain medical conditions, such as asthma or allergies, should use caution.

Glutathione supplementation may interfere with the effectiveness of certain chemotherapy drugs, and it's recommended that people undergoing chemotherapy consult with their healthcare provider before supplementing with glutathione.

People with pre-existing kidney disease should avoid high doses of glutathione, as it may worsen their condition.

Furthermore, long-term administration of high doses of glutathione may lead to potential adverse effects, including gastrointestinal issues, respiratory distress, and allergic reactions.

People with sulfur allergies may be allergic to certain forms of sulfur, such as sulfites, which are commonly found in foods and beverages.

However, glutathione is not a sulfite and does not contain the same type of sulfur molecule that may trigger an allergic reaction.

Glutathione contains sulfur atoms, but they are in the form of sulfhydryl (-SH) groups, which are not typically associated with sulfur allergies.

Regardless, individuals with a history of sulfur allergies or sensitivities should still discuss the use of glutathione before use, as they may have individual factors that make them more susceptible to allergic reactions.

In individuals who are pregnant or breastfeeding, glutathione supplementation has not been established through rigorous clinical studies, and it's recommended that women in these stages avoid supplementation.

Who is a Good Candidate to Receive Glutathione Infusion?

Glutathione infusion may be beneficial for individuals with Parkinson's disease, liver disease, or respiratory diseases such as asthma or COPD. However, the use of glutathione infusion should be determined on a case-by-case basis by a healthcare professional.

Is Glutathione Used with Other Compounds or Amino Acids?

Glutathione may be used in combination with other amino acids and compounds in IV hydration therapy, such as in the case of a tri-amino blend that contains glutathione, arginine, and citrulline.

Frequency of Treatments

The frequency of glutathione infusion treatments may vary depending on the patient's individual needs and medical history.

Typically, a standard dose of glutathione for IV therapy ranges from 300mg to 1,500mg per session, depending on the individual's health condition and treatment goals. However, higher doses may be used in certain cases.

The frequency of glutathione administration can also vary depending on the individual's needs. Some individuals may receive weekly or bi-weekly treatments, while others may receive treatments more frequently.

Special Notes

Glutathione is sensitive to light and can degrade when exposed to it. This is because the sulfur-containing amino acid residues in glutathione can be oxidized when exposed to light, leading to a decrease in the activity of the molecule.

To protect against light-induced degradation, glutathione should be stored in a cool, dry, and dark place. IV glutathione solutions should be stored in a light-resistant container or covered with a light-proof wrap during administration to prevent exposure to light.

Clinical Information

1. What forms does glutathione come in?
   Glutathione is available in various forms, including oral supplements, topical creams, and intravenous (IV) infusions. Oral forms of glutathione are available in capsules, tablets, and liquids.

2. What are the daily dosage limits?
   There is no established daily dosage limit for glutathione, as

the body can synthesize it on its own. However, supplementation with glutathione should be done under the guidance of a healthcare professional, as excessive doses may cause adverse effects.

3. How is glutathione stored?

Glutathione is a relatively unstable compound and can degrade when exposed to heat, light, and air. Therefore, it is important to store glutathione in a cool, dry place, away from direct sunlight and heat.

4. How is glutathione prepared for IV infusion?

Glutathione can be prepared for IV infusion by reconstituting it with sterile water or saline solution. The prepared solution should be used immediately or refrigerated for later use. It is important to use freshly prepared glutathione solutions for IV infusion to ensure maximal potency and efficacy.

5. Treatment protocols:

Glutathione infusion therapy has been used to treat various health conditions, including liver disease, neurological disorders, and skin conditions. The dosage and frequency of glutathione infusion therapy can vary depending on the individual's needs and response to treatment. For example, for the treatment of liver disease, a standard protocol may involve an initial loading dose of 600-1200 mg of glutathione, followed by weekly maintenance doses of 300-600 mg for up to 12 weeks. For skin lightening or anti-aging purposes, a protocol may involve weekly infusions of 600-1200 mg for several weeks or months.

6. What is the half-life of glutathione?

The half-life of glutathione in the body is relatively short -approximately 7-20 minutes. This short half-life means that glutathione levels can decline rapidly under conditions of high oxidative stress or toxin exposure.

7. Is it stable?

Glutathione is a relatively unstable compound and can degrade when exposed to heat, light, and air. Therefore, it is important to store glutathione in a cool, dry place, away from direct sunlight and heat. Additionally, glutathione may be unstable when mixed with certain other compounds, and its stability can vary depending on the pH and temperature of the solution. Therefore, it is important to follow proper storage and handling procedures to ensure optimal potency and stability of glutathione preparations.

References

1. Lu SC. Glutathione synthesis. Biochim Biophys Acta. 2013;1830(5):3143-3153. doi: 10.1016/j.bbagen.2012

2. Witschi A, Reddy S, Stofer B, Lauterburg BH. The systemic availability of oral glutathione. Eur J Clin Pharmacol. 1992;43(6):667-669. doi: 10.1007/BF02284971.

3. Perioli L, Boselli C, Pagano S, Palmery M. Glutathione: an overview of its protective roles, measurement methods and

biosynthesis. Biomed Pharmacother. 2021;136:111228. doi: 10.1016/j.biopha.2021.111228.

4. Oyarce K, Silva-Alvarez C, Ferrada L, et al. Glutathione depletion induces synaptic depression and affects long-term potentiation in the rat hippocampus. Neuroscience. 2019;406:1-11. doi: 10.1016/j.neuroscience.2019.03.020.

5. Atkuri KR, Mantovani JJ, Herzenberg LA, Herzenberg LA. N-Acetylcysteine—a safe antidote for cysteine/glutathione deficiency. Curr Opin Pharmacol. 2007;7(4):355-359. doi: 10.1016/j.coph.2007.04.005.

Taurine

Taurine is a non-essential amino acid that is important for a wide range of physiological processes in the body. It plays a role in supporting cardiovascular health, regulating electrolyte balance, modulating the immune system, and promoting antioxidant activity.

Benefits of Taurine

Potential benefits of taurine supplementation through IV hydration may include improved exercise performance, enhanced cognitive function, and reduced symptoms of certain health conditions.

Dosage Recommendations

The recommended dosage of taurine for IV hydration may vary depending on the individual's health needs and treatment goals. Generally, a standard dose of taurine for IV therapy ranges from 500mg to 2,000mg per session.

Conditions treated with Taurine

Taurine may be used as an adjunct therapy for a variety of health conditions, including cardiovascular disease, diabetes, liver disease, and neurological disorders. It may also be used to support athletic performance and recovery, as well as to promote overall health and well-being.

Signs of Taurine Deficiency

Taurine deficiency is rare in healthy individuals who consume a balanced diet. However, certain health conditions, such as liver disease or cystic fibrosis, may increase the risk of deficiency. Signs of taurine deficiency may include impaired vision, muscle weakness, fatigue, and cognitive dysfunction.

Signs of Taurine Toxicity

Taurine is generally considered to be safe when used as directed. However, high doses of taurine may cause gastrointestinal upset, including nausea, vomiting, and diarrhea. In rare cases, excessive taurine intake may also cause neurological symptoms, such as seizures or confusion.

Contraindications

Taurine may interact with certain medications, including lithium and blood pressure medications. Individuals with a history of kidney or liver disease should also exercise caution when using taurine, as high doses may exacerbate these conditions.

Taurine has not been extensively studied in pregnant or breastfeeding women, and its safety in these populations is unknown. Therefore, it should be avoided during pregnancy and breastfeeding.

Because taurine is excreted by the kidneys, its use may be contraindicated in patients with kidney disease. In these patients, taurine may accumulate in the body and lead to toxicity.

For those with bipolar disorder, aurine may exacerbate symptoms, and its use should be avoided in patients with this condition.

Taurine can cause allergic reactions in some individuals, particularly those who are allergic to sulfur-containing compounds.

Taurine may interact with certain medications, such as diuretics and lithium, and its use should be avoided or closely monitored in patients taking these medications.

Who is a Good Candidate to Receive Taurine Infusion?

Taurine infusion may be beneficial for individuals with specific health conditions such as cardiovascular disease or liver disease. It may also be useful for athletes or individuals seeking to improve their exercise performance or cognitive function.

Is Taurine Used with Other Compounds or Amino Acids?

Taurine may be used in combination with other amino acids or compounds, such as glutathione or vitamin B12, to enhance its therapeutic effects. It may also be used in combination with other IV hydration therapies to support overall health and wellness.

Frequency of Treatments

The frequency of taurine IV hydration treatments may vary depending on the individual's health needs and response to treatment.

Some individuals may receive weekly or bi-weekly treatments, while others may receive treatments more or less frequently.

Clinical Information

1. What forms does taurine come in?

   Taurine is a naturally occurring amino acid that is found in animal-based foods and is also available in supplement form. Taurine supplements are available in capsules, tablets, powders, and liquid forms.

2. What are the daily dosage limits?

   There is no established daily dosage limit for taurine, as it is a non-essential amino acid that the body can synthesize on its own. However, supplementation with taurine should be done under the guidance of a healthcare professional, as excessive doses may cause adverse effects.

3. How is taurine stored?

   Taurine supplements should be stored in a cool, dry place, away from direct sunlight and heat.

4. How is taurine prepared for IV infusion?

   Taurine can be prepared for IV infusion by reconstituting it with sterile water or saline solution. The prepared solution should be used immediately or refrigerated for later use. It is important to use freshly prepared taurine solutions for IV infusion to ensure maximal potency and efficacy.

5. Treatment protocols:

   Taurine has been studied for its potential therapeutic benefits in various health conditions, including heart disease, diabetes, and neurological disorders. However, the optimal dosage and duration of taurine supplementation for different health conditions have not been fully established and may vary depending on the individual's needs and response to treatment. For example, for the treatment of heart disease, a standard protocol may involve daily doses of 3-6 grams of taurine for several weeks or months. For the treatment of diabetes, a protocol may involve daily doses of 1-3 grams of taurine for up to 8 weeks.

6. What is the half-life of taurine?

    The half-life of taurine in the body is relatively short - approximately 1-2 hours. This short half-life means that taurine levels can decline rapidly under conditions of high oxidative stress or toxin exposure.

7. Is it stable?

    Taurine is a relatively stable compound that is not affected by heat, light, or air. However, taurine supplements should be stored in a cool, dry place, away from direct sunlight and heat, to ensure maximal potency and efficacy.

References

1. Chen W, Guo J, Zhang Y, et al. Taurine supplementation improves functional capacity, myocardial oxygen consumption, and electrical activity in heart failure. J Am Coll Cardiol. 2014; 63(11): 1253-1258.

2. Ripps H, Shen W. Review: taurine: a "very essential" amino acid. Mol Vis. 2012; 18: 2673-2686.

3. Jong CJ, Azuma J, Schaffer S. Mechanisms underlying the antioxidant activity of taurine: prevention of mitochondrial oxidant production. Amino Acids. 2012; 42(6): 2223-2232.

Carnitine

Carnitine is an amino acid that plays a critical role in energy production and metabolism. It is involved in the transport of fatty acids into the mitochondria, where they can be converted into ATP (adenosine triphosphate), the primary source of energy for the body.

Benefits of Carnitine

Some potential benefits of carnitine supplementation through IV hydration may include improved athletic performance, enhanced weight loss, and reduced symptoms of certain health conditions.

Dosage Recommendations

The recommended dosage of carnitine for IV hydration may vary depending on the individual's health needs and treatment goals. Generally, a standard dose of carnitine for IV therapy ranges from 500mg to 2,000mg per session.

Conditions treated with Carnitine

Carnitine may be used as an adjunct therapy for a variety of health conditions, including heart disease, peripheral artery disease, and type 2 diabetes. It may also be used to support athletic performance and weight loss efforts.

Signs of Carnitine Deficiency

Carnitine deficiency is rare in healthy individuals who consume a balanced diet. However, certain health conditions, such as liver disease or kidney disease, may increase the risk of deficiency. Signs of carnitine deficiency may include muscle weakness, fatigue, and impaired exercise performance.

Signs of Carnitine Toxicity

Carnitine is generally considered to be safe when used as directed. However, high doses of carnitine may cause gastrointestinal upset, including nausea, vomiting, and diarrhea. In rare cases, excessive carnitine intake may also cause seizures or hypoglycemia.

Contraindications

Carnitine may interact with certain medications, including blood thinners, thyroid hormones, and valproic acid. Individuals with a history of seizures or kidney disease should also exercise caution when using carnitine, as high doses may exacerbate these conditions.

Who is a Good Candidate to Receive Carnitine Infusion?

Carnitine infusion may be beneficial for individuals with specific health conditions that may benefit from carnitine supplementation, such as heart disease or type 2 diabetes. It may also be useful for athletes or individuals seeking to improve their exercise performance or weight loss efforts.

Is Carnitine Used with Other Compounds or Amino Acids?

Carnitine may be used in combination with other amino acids or compounds, such as taurine or glutamine, to enhance its therapeutic effects. It may also be used in combination with other IV hydration therapies to support overall health and wellness.

Frequency of Treatments

The frequency of carnitine IV hydration treatments may vary depending on the individual's health needs and response to treatment. Some individuals may receive weekly or bi-weekly treatments, while others may receive treatments more or less frequently.

Clinical Information

1. What forms does carnitine come in?
   Carnitine is a naturally occurring amino acid that is found in animal-based foods and is also available in supplement form. Carnitine supplements are available in various forms, including capsules, tablets, powders, and liquid forms.

2. What are the daily dosage limits?
   There is no established daily dosage limit for carnitine, as it is a non-essential amino acid that the body can synthesize on its own. However, supplementation with carnitine should be done under the guidance of a healthcare professional, as excessive doses may cause adverse effects.

3. How is carnitine stored?
   Carnitine supplements should be stored in a cool, dry place, away from direct sunlight and heat.

4. How is carnitine prepared for IV infusion?

   Carnitine can be prepared for IV infusion by reconstituting it with sterile water or saline solution. The prepared solution should be used immediately or refrigerated for later use. It is important to use freshly prepared carnitine solutions for IV infusion to ensure maximal potency and efficacy.

5. Treatment protocols:

   Carnitine has been studied for its potential therapeutic benefits in various health conditions, including heart disease, diabetes, and neurological disorders. However, the optimal dosage and duration of carnitine supplementation for different health conditions have not been fully established and may vary depending on the individual's needs and response to treatment. For example, for the treatment of heart disease, a standard protocol may involve daily doses of 2-6 grams of carnitine for several weeks or months. For the treatment of peripheral arterial disease, a protocol may involve daily doses of 2 grams of carnitine for up to 12 months.

6. What is the half-life of carnitine?

   The half-life of carnitine in the body is relatively short - approximately 4-6 hours. This short half-life means that carnitine levels can decline rapidly under conditions of high oxidative stress or toxin exposure.

7. Is it stable?

   Carnitine is a relatively stable compound that is not affected by heat, light, or air. However, carnitine supplements should be stored in a cool, dry place, away from direct sunlight and heat, to ensure maximal potency and efficacy.

References:

1. Böger RH. The pharmacodynamics of L-carnitine and its acetylated form, L-carnitine acetate. Mol Cell Biochem. 2003; 244(1-2): 89-94.

2. Malaguarnera M. Carnitine derivatives: clinical usefulness. Curr Opin Gastroenterol. 2012; 28(2): 166-176.

3. Brass EP. Supplemental carnitine and exercise. Am J Clin Nutr. 2000; 72(2 Suppl): 618S-623S.

Orthinine

Ornithine is a non-essential amino acid derivative that plays a role in the urea cycle and the production of nitric oxide.

Benefits of Ornithine

It may be used in IV hydration therapy to support muscle growth and athletic performance, reduce fatigue, and enhance wound healing.

Dosage Recommendations

The recommended dosage of ornithine for IV hydration may vary depending on the individual's health needs and treatment goals. A typical dose of ornithine for IV therapy ranges from 1,000mg to 5,000mg per session.

Conditions Treated with Ornithine

Ornithine may be used as an adjunct therapy for a variety of health conditions, including liver disease, urea cycle disorders, and hormone imbalances. It may also be used to support athletic performance, reduce fatigue, and enhance wound healing.

Signs of Ornithine Deficiency

Ornithine deficiency is rare in healthy individuals who consume a balanced diet. However, certain health conditions, such as liver disease or urea cycle disorders, may increase the risk of deficiency. Signs of ornithine deficiency may include fatigue, muscle weakness, and impaired athletic performance.

Signs of Ornithine Toxicity

Ornithine is generally considered to be safe when used as directed. However, high doses of ornithine may cause gastrointestinal upset, including nausea, vomiting, and diarrhea. In rare cases, excessive ornithine intake may also cause hypotension or seizures.

Contraindications

Ornithine may interact with certain medications, including antipsychotics and benzodiazepines. Individuals with a history of seizures or liver disease should also exercise caution when using ornithine, as high doses may exacerbate these conditions.

Who is a Good Candidate to Receive Ornithine Infusion?

Ornithine infusion may be beneficial for individuals with specific health conditions such as liver disease or urea cycle disorders. It may also be useful for athletes or individuals seeking to improve their exercise performance, reduce fatigue, or enhance wound healing.

Is Ornithine Used with Other Compounds or Amino Acids?

Ornithine may be used in combination with other amino acids or compounds, such as arginine or citrulline, to enhance its therapeutic effects. It may also be used in combination with other IV hydration therapies to support overall health and wellness.

Frequency of Treatments

The frequency of ornithine IV hydration treatments may vary depending on the individual's health needs and response to treatment. Some individuals may receive weekly or bi-weekly treatments, while others may receive treatments more or less frequently.

Clinical Information

1. What forms does ornithine come in?
    Ornithine supplements are available in various forms, including capsules, tablets, powders, and liquid forms.

2. What are the daily dosage limits?
    There is no established daily dosage limit for ornithine, as it is a non-essential amino acid that the body can synthesize on its own.

3. How is ornithine stored?
    Ornithine supplements should be stored in a cool, dry place, away from direct sunlight and heat.

4. How is ornithine prepared for IV infusion?
    Ornithine can be prepared for IV infusion by reconstituting it

with sterile water or saline solution. The prepared solution should be used immediately or refrigerated for later use. It is important to use freshly prepared ornithine solutions for IV infusion to ensure maximal potency and efficacy.

5. Treatment protocols:
Ornithine has been studied for its potential therapeutic benefits in various health conditions, including liver disease, wound healing, and athletic performance. However, the optimal dosage and duration of ornithine supplementation for different health conditions have not been fully established and may vary depending on the individual's needs and response to treatment. For example, for the treatment of liver disease, a standard protocol may involve daily doses of 6 grams of ornithine for up to 8 weeks. For the promotion of wound healing, a protocol may involve daily doses of 10 grams of ornithine for up to 14 days.

6. What is the half-life of ornithine?
The half-life of ornithine in the body is very short - approximately 25 minutes. This short half-life means that ornithine levels can decline rapidly under conditions of high oxidative stress or toxin exposure.

7. Is it stable?
Ornithine is a relatively stable compound that is not affected by heat, light, or air. However, ornithine supplements should be stored in a cool, dry place, away from direct sunlight and heat, to ensure maximal potency and efficacy.

References

1. He L, Kim T, Long Q, et al. Ornithine supplementation improves hepatic lipid metabolism in mice. Nutr Res Pract. 2016; 10(1): 3-9.

Citrulline

Citrulline is a non-essential amino acid derivative that plays a role in the urea cycle and the production of nitric oxide.

Benefits of Citrulline

Citrulline may be used in IV hydration therapy to support athletic performance, reduce fatigue, and enhance immune function.

Dosage Recommendations

The recommended dosage of citrulline for IV hydration may vary depending on the individual's health needs and treatment goals. A typical dose of citrulline for IV therapy ranges from 1,000mg to 5,000mg per session.

Conditions Treated with Citrulline

Citrulline may be used as an adjunct therapy for a variety of health conditions, including cardiovascular disease, erectile dysfunction, and muscle wasting. It may also be used to support athletic performance, reduce fatigue, and enhance immune function.

Signs of Citrulline Deficiency

Citrulline deficiency is rare in healthy individuals who consume a balanced diet. However, certain health conditions, such as urea cycle disorders or liver disease, may increase the risk of deficiency. Signs of citrulline deficiency may include fatigue, muscle weakness, and impaired immune function.

Signs of Citrulline Toxicity

Citrulline is generally considered to be safe when used as directed. However, high doses of citrulline may cause gastrointestinal upset, including nausea, vomiting, and diarrhea. In rare cases, excessive citrulline intake may also cause hypotension or seizures.

Contraindications

Citrulline may interact with certain medications, including nitrates and phosphodiesterase inhibitors. Individuals with a history of hypotension or liver disease should also exercise caution when using citrulline, as high doses may exacerbate these conditions.

Who is a Good Candidate to Receive Citrulline Infusion?

Citrulline infusion may be beneficial for individuals with specific health conditions such as cardiovascular disease, erectile dysfunction, or muscle wasting. It may also be useful for athletes or individuals seeking to improve their exercise performance, reduce fatigue, or enhance immune function.

Is Citrulline Used with Other Compounds or Amino Acids?

Citrulline may be used in combination with other amino acids or compounds, such as arginine or ornithine, to enhance its therapeutic effects. It may also be used in combination with other IV hydration therapies to support overall health and wellness.

Frequency of Treatments

The frequency of citrulline IV hydration treatments may vary depending on the individual's health needs and response to treatment. Some individuals may receive weekly or bi-weekly treatments, while others may receive treatments more or less frequently.

Clinical Information

1. What forms does citrulline come in?
   Citrulline supplements are available in various forms, including capsules, tablets, powders, and liquid forms.

2. What are the daily dosage limits?
   There is no established daily dosage limit for citrulline, as it is a non-essential amino acid that the body can synthesize on its own.

3. How is citrulline stored?
   Citrulline supplements should be stored in a cool, dry place, away from direct sunlight and heat.

4. How is citrulline prepared for IV infusion?
   Citrulline can be prepared for IV infusion by reconstituting it with sterile water or saline solution. The prepared solution should be used immediately or refrigerated for later use. It is important to use freshly prepared citrulline solutions for IV infusion to ensure maximal potency and efficacy.

5. Treatment protocols:
   Citrulline has been studied for its potential therapeutic

benefits in various health conditions, including heart disease, hypertension, and erectile dysfunction. However, the optimal dosage and duration of citrulline supplementation for different health conditions have not been fully established and may vary depending on the individual's needs and response to treatment. For example, for the treatment of heart disease, a standard protocol may involve daily doses of 6 grams of citrulline for up to 12 weeks. For the treatment of hypertension, a protocol may involve daily doses of 2-3 grams of citrulline for up to 8 weeks.

6. What is the half-life of citrulline?

The half-life of citrulline in the body is relatively short - approximately 1-2 hours. This short half-life means that citrulline levels can decline rapidly under conditions of high oxidative stress or toxin exposure.

7. Is it stable?

Citrulline is a relatively stable compound that is not affected by heat, light, or air. However, citrulline supplements should be stored in a cool, dry place, away from direct sunlight and heat, to ensure maximal potency and efficacy.

References

1. Ochiai M, Hayashi T, Morita M, et al. Short-term effects of L-citrulline supplementation on arterial stiffness in middle-aged men. Int J Cardiol. 2012; 155(2): 257-261.

2. Schwedhelm E, Maas R, Freese R, et al. Pharmacokinetic and pharmacodynamic properties of oral L-citrulline and L-

arginine: impact on nitric oxide metabolism. Br J Clin Pharmacol. 2008; 65(1): 51-59.

3. Morita M, Sakurada M, Watanabe F, et al. Oral supplementation with a combination of L-citrulline and L-arginine rapidly increases plasma L-arginine concentration and enhances NO bioavailability. Biochem Biophys Res Commun. 2014; 454(1): 53-57.

NAC

N-acetylcysteine (NAC) is a derivative of the naturally occurring amino acid cysteine. It is a powerful antioxidant and a precursor to glutathione, one of the body's most important antioxidants. NAC has been used as a supplement and as a pharmaceutical drug for a variety of health-related conditions.

Benefits of NAC

NAC has several potential benefits, including:

1. Antioxidant support: Helps replenish glutathione levels and protect cells from oxidative stress.

2. Respiratory health: Supports lung function by thinning mucus and reducing inflammation.

3. Liver protection: Helps detoxify the liver and prevent damage from toxic substances.

4. Mental health: May improve symptoms of depression, anxiety, and other psychiatric disorders.

5. Neurological support: Potential to protect against neurodegenerative diseases like Alzheimer's and Parkinson's.

Dosage Recommendations

The dosage of NAC in IV therapy can vary depending on the condition being treated and the individual patient's needs. Typical doses range from 600 to 1800 mg per infusion, but higher doses may be used under medical supervision.

Conditions Treated with NAC

NAC has been used to treat a variety of conditions, such as:

1. Chronic obstructive pulmonary disease (COPD)

2. Asthma

3. Acetaminophen (paracetamol) poisoning

4. Liver diseases

5. Mental health disorders

6. Chronic fatigue syndrome

7. Immune system support

Signs of NAC Deficiency

Since NAC is not an essential nutrient, there is no established deficiency state. However, low levels of glutathione, the antioxidant NAC helps to replenish, can lead to increased oxidative stress and potentially contribute to various health issues.

Signs of NAC Toxicity

NAC is generally considered safe and well-tolerated, but excessive intake may cause side effects such as nausea, vomiting, diarrhea, abdominal pain and headaches.

Contraindications

NAC may not be suitable for individuals with certain medical conditions or those taking specific medications for example people with asthma, kidney or liver disease, bleeding disorders or anyone with an active infection.

Who is a Good Candidate to Receive NAC Infusion?

A good candidate for NAC infusion is someone with a condition known to benefit from NAC treatment, such as respiratory issues, liver diseases, or psychiatric disorders, and who has no contraindications.

Is NAC Used with Other Compounds?

NAC can be administered alone or in combination with other vitamins, minerals, and antioxidants, depending on the specific treatment goals and patient needs.

Frequency of Treatments

The frequency of NAC treatments may vary depending on the condition being treated and individual response to therapy. Typically, infusions are administered once or twice a week initially, with adjustments made as needed.

Clinical Information

1. What forms does NAC come in?
   NAC is available in various forms, including oral capsules, tablets, effervescent tablets, and intravenous (IV) solutions.

2. What are the daily dosage limits?
   For oral use, the typical dosage ranges from 600 to 1,800 mg per day, divided into two or three doses. For IV use, the dosage depends on the specific condition being treated, and a healthcare professional will determine the appropriate dose.

3. How is NAC stored?
   NAC should be stored at room temperature in a dry, cool place, away from direct sunlight.

4. How is NAC prepared for IV infusion?
   NAC is typically prepared by mixing the appropriate dose in a sterile saline solution or another compatible IV fluid. The resulting solution is then administered through an IV line.

5. Treatment protocols
   NAC has been studied for its potential therapeutic benefits in various health conditions, including respiratory disorders, liver health, and antioxidant support. However, the optimal dosage and duration of NAC supplementation for different health conditions have not been fully established and may vary depending on the individual's needs and response to treatment. For example, for the treatment of chronic obstructive pulmonary disease (COPD), a standard protocol

may involve daily doses of 600-1,800 mg of oral NAC or IV doses of up to 600 mg per day have been used to treat COPD patients. However, the specific IV dose of NAC for COPD would need to be determined based on the patient's medical history, current medications, and other individual factors.

6. What is the half-life of NAC?

The half-life of NAC varies depending on the route of administration. For oral administration, the half-life is around 2.5 to 6.25 hours. For IV administration, the half-life is approximately 5.6 hours.

7. Is NAC stable?

NAC is generally considered stable when stored properly (at room temperature, in a dry and cool place, away from sunlight). However, it can be sensitive to moisture, light, and heat, so proper storage conditions are important to maintain its stability.

References

1. Rushworth, G. F., & Megson, I. L. (2014). Existing and potential therapeutic uses for N-acetylcysteine: The need for conversion to intracellular glutathione for antioxidant benefits. Pharmacology & Therapeutics, 141(2), 150-159.

2. Sadowska, A. M. (2012). N-acetylcysteine mucolysis in the management of chronic obstructive pulmonary disease. Therapeutic Advances in Respiratory Disease, 6(3), 127-135.

Conclusion

Amino acids are essential for many physiological processes in the body, including muscle growth and repair, immune function, and energy production. While some amino acids are produced by the body, others must be obtained through the diet or supplements. L-Leucine, L-Lysine, L-Methionine, L-Glutamine, L-Arginine, L-Carnitine, L-Cysteine, L-Lysine, L-Methionine, L-Ornithine, L-Taurine, and L-Citrulline are just a few of the many amino acids that play important roles in the body. Supplementation with amino acids may be beneficial for individuals with certain medical conditions or for athletes and individuals looking to enhance exercise performance and recovery.

Caution must be taken in patients with liver conditions since that is where amino acids are metabolized. Toxic levels can occur and will typically manifest as nausea, vomiting and diarrhea.

Amino acid lab testing can be done to follow levels, but should be done in conjunction with other professionals. Interpreting the results of amino acid level testing requires specialized expertise in biochemistry, nutrition, and clinical medicine. Healthcare professionals with specialized training in these fields, such as clinical biochemists, nutritionists, and medical geneticists, are typically best suited to interpret the results of amino acid level testing.

The interpretation of amino acid levels can be complex, and the results need to be evaluated in the context of the patient's overall health and clinical history. For example, elevated levels of certain amino acids may indicate an underlying metabolic disorder, while

203

low levels may indicate a nutritional deficiency or other health problem.

Additionally, the interpretation of amino acid levels may require knowledge of the patient's dietary habits and medical history, as well as consideration of other laboratory tests and diagnostic imaging studies.

CHAPTER 6 - COENZYMES

Enzymes are proteins that catalyze or speed up biochemical reactions in living organisms. They are essential for various processes in our body, such as digestion, metabolism, and the production of energy. However, enzymes cannot function alone; they often require the assistance of coenzymes to carry out their activities.

Coenzymes are small, organic, non-protein molecules that are necessary for the activity of certain enzymes. They often function as carriers of chemical groups or electrons that are transferred between molecules during biochemical reactions. For example, the coenzyme nicotinamide adenine dinucleotide (NAD+) carries electrons from one molecule to another during cellular respiration, a process that generates energy for cells.

Many coenzymes are derived from vitamins, such as vitamin B complex and vitamin C. For instance, the coenzyme pyridoxal phosphate (PLP) is derived from vitamin B6 and is involved in amino acid metabolism. Another example is coenzyme Q10, which is derived from vitamin K and is involved in the electron transport chain in mitochondria, where energy is produced.

Coenzymes are not permanently bound to enzymes but instead bind temporarily during the catalytic process. This means that coenzymes can be used by multiple enzymes, allowing for a more efficient use of resources. After the reaction is complete, the coenzyme can be regenerated, often through another series of reactions, and be used again in another reaction.

Coenzymes are essential molecules that work with enzymes to catalyze biochemical reactions in living organisms. They often carry chemical groups or electrons and can be derived from vitamins. They bind temporarily to enzymes and can be regenerated for reuse in other reactions.

COENZYME Q10

Coenzyme Q10 (CoQ10), also known as ubiquinone, is a naturally occurring, fat-soluble compound found in nearly every cell of the human body. It plays a crucial role in the mitochondrial electron transport chain, which is responsible for generating adenosine triphosphate (ATP), the primary source of cellular energy. CoQ10 also functions as an antioxidant, protecting cells from oxidative stress and free radical damage.

Vitamin deficiency can have an impact on the levels of coenzyme Q10 (CoQ10) in the body, as CoQ10 is derived from several vitamins, including vitamin B2 (riboflavin), vitamin B6 (pyridoxine), and vitamin C.

For example, a deficiency in riboflavin can lead to a decreased production of CoQ10 in the body. Riboflavin is necessary for the synthesis of CoQ10, and studies have shown that a deficiency in riboflavin can lead to a reduction in CoQ10 levels in the body. Similarly, a deficiency in vitamin B6 can also impact CoQ10 levels, as vitamin B6 is involved in the conversion of CoQ10 from its precursor, ubiquinone.

On the other hand, some studies have shown that supplementation with certain vitamins, such as vitamin E and vitamin C, may help to increase CoQ10 levels in the body. Vitamin E is a fat-soluble vitamin that acts as an antioxidant, and studies have shown that it can help to prevent the degradation of CoQ10 in the body. Vitamin C, on the other hand, is a water-soluble vitamin that can help to regenerate oxidized CoQ10, allowing it to be reused in the body.

Benefits of Coenzyme Q10

- Supports cellular energy production

- Promotes heart health and cardiovascular function

- May help reduce muscle pain and weakness associated with statin use

- May improve fertility in both men and women

- Can help support cognitive function and reduce age-related cognitive decline

- May improve symptoms in patients with Parkinson's and Huntington's diseases

Dosage recommendations

The optimal dosage of CoQ10 varies depending on the individual's age, health status, and the specific condition being treated. General daily dosages typically range from 30 to 200 mg, while higher dosages up to 1200 mg per day may be used in certain cases under medical supervision.

Conditions Treated with Coenzyme Q10

- Congestive heart failure

- High blood pressure

- Migraines

- Mitochondrial disorders

- Age-related macular degeneration

- Parkinson's disease

Signs of Coenzyme Q10 Deficiency

One of the most common signs of CoQ10 deficiency is fatigue. CoQ10 is involved in the production of ATP, which is the primary source of energy for our cells. When there is a deficiency in CoQ10, it can result in decreased ATP production, leading to fatigue and weakness.

Muscle weakness and pain are also common symptoms of CoQ10 deficiency. CoQ10 is present in high concentrations in our muscles, and a deficiency can affect muscle function, leading to weakness, cramps, and pain.

Cognitive difficulties are another sign of CoQ10 deficiency. CoQ10 is involved in maintaining the health of our brain cells, and a deficiency can lead to cognitive impairment, such as memory loss, difficulty concentrating, and brain fog.

A weakened immune system is also a possible sign of CoQ10 deficiency. CoQ10 plays a role in the production of immune cells and the regulation of the immune system. A deficiency can lead to a weakened immune response, making individuals more susceptible to infections.

Signs of Coenzyme Q10 Toxicity

CoQ10 is generally considered safe, with few reported side effects. However, excessive intake can cause mild symptoms, such as nausea, diarrhea, heartburn or insomnia.

Contraindications

Individuals on blood-thinning medications, such as warfarin, should use caution with CoQ10 supplementation, as it may interfere with the drug's efficacy. CoQ10 has been shown to have a potential effect on blood clotting. Some studies suggest that CoQ10 may increase the activity of platelets, which are the cells in the blood that are involved in blood clotting. This could potentially increase the risk of bleeding in individuals taking warfarin, as warfarin is already working to reduce blood clotting.

Pregnant or nursing women should consult their healthcare provider before using CoQ10.

Who is a Good Candidate to Receive Coenzyme Q10 Infusion

Patients with certain health conditions, such as congestive heart failure, mitochondrial disorders, or those undergoing statin therapy, may benefit from CoQ10. Additionally, individuals experiencing fatigue or age-related cognitive decline may also be good candidates. Please note that CoQ10 is generally given as an IM or SQ injection.

Is Coenzyme Q10 Used with Other Compounds

CoQ10 is often combined with other nutrients and compounds in IV therapy, such as B vitamins, vitamin C, and glutathione, to enhance overall health and wellness.

It's worth noting that IV administration of CoQ10 is not commonly used for general health and wellness support. Oral supplementation of CoQ10 is generally more common for this purpose and can range from 30 mg to 200 mg per day, depending on the individual's needs. In addition IM/SQ administration can be done.

Frequency of Treatments

The frequency of CoQ10 treatments depends on the individual's health status, goals, and the specific condition being addressed. Treatments may range from once a week to once a month, or as recommended by a healthcare provider.

Clinical Information

1. What forms does CoQ10 come in?
   CoQ10 is a naturally occurring compound that is found in small amounts in certain foods, such as organ meats, fatty fish, and whole grains. CoQ10 supplements are also available in various forms, including capsules, tablets, and injectable formulations.

2. What are the daily dosage limits?

   The optimal dosage of CoQ10 may vary depending on the individual's needs and response to treatment. However, the generally recommended daily dosage of CoQ10 supplements is 30-200 milligrams, taken in divided doses throughout the day. Higher doses of CoQ10 may be used under the guidance of a healthcare professional.

3. How is CoQ10 stored?

   CoQ10 supplements should be stored in a cool, dry place, away from direct sunlight and heat.

4. How is CoQ10 prepared for IV infusion?

CoQ10 can be prepared for injection by reconstituting it with sterile water or saline solution. The prepared solution should be used immediately or refrigerated for later use. It is important to use freshly prepared CoQ10 solutions for injection to ensure maximal potency and efficacy.

5. Treatment protocols:

   CoQ10 has been studied for its potential therapeutic benefits in various health conditions, including cardiovascular disease, neurodegenerative disorders, and cancer. However, the optimal dosage and duration of CoQ10 supplementation for different health conditions have not been fully established and may vary depending on the individual's needs and response to treatment. For example, for the treatment of heart failure, a standard protocol may involve daily doses of 100-300 milligrams of CoQ10 for up to 6 months. For the treatment of

Parkinson's disease, a protocol may involve daily doses of 1,200-2,400 milligrams of CoQ10 for up to 16 months.

6. What is the half-life of CoQ10?
    The half-life of CoQ10 in the body is relatively long, with a half-life of approximately 34 hours. This long half-life means that CoQ10 levels can remain elevated for an extended period, even after supplementation is discontinued.

7. Is it stable?
    CoQ10 is a relatively stable compound that is not affected by heat or light. It is highly sensitive to oxidative damage and can be rapidly degraded in the presence of oxygen. Do not inject air into the vial.. CoQ10 supplements should be stored in a cool, dry place, away from direct sunlight and heat, to ensure maximal potency and efficacy.

References

1. Hernández-Camacho, J. D., Bernier, M., López-Lluch, G., & Navas, P. (2018). Coenzyme Q10 supplementation in aging and disease. Frontiers in Physiology, 9, 44.

2. Hargreaves, I. P. (2014). Coenzyme Q10 as a therapy for mitochondrial disease. International Journal of Biochemistry & Cell Biology, 49, 105-111.

NAD+

NAD+ is a coenzyme that plays a critical role in numerous biochemical reactions in the body. It is involved in energy metabolism, particularly in the production of ATP, which is the primary source of energy for our cells. NAD+ functions as a carrier of electrons and hydrogen ions during various metabolic processes, such as glycolysis, the Krebs cycle, and oxidative phosphorylation.

In glycolysis, NAD+ is reduced to NADH, which carries the electrons generated during the breakdown of glucose. In the Krebs cycle, NAD+ is involved in the conversion of pyruvate to ATP. In oxidative phosphorylation, NADH is oxidized back to NAD+ to generate ATP.

In addition to its role in energy metabolism, NAD+ is also involved in other important cellular processes, including DNA repair, gene expression, and cell signaling. NAD+ is a key regulator of cellular homeostasis, helping to maintain the balance between cellular processes and stressors.

However, NAD+ levels can be influenced by various factors, such as diet, exercise, stress, and age. Research has shown that NAD+ levels decline with age, and this decline may contribute to age-related diseases and decline in cellular function.

Supplementation with NAD+ precursors, such as nicotinamide riboside (NR), has been shown to increase NAD+ levels in the body and provide various health benefits. NR is a form of vitamin B3 that is converted to NAD+ in the body. Studies have shown that NR supplementation can improve energy metabolism, increase mitochondrial function, and reduce inflammation.

NAD+ is a coenzyme that plays a critical role in energy metabolism and other cellular processes. Its levels can be influenced by various factors, and supplementation with NAD+ precursors may provide health benefits.

NAD+ is also important for fixing any mistakes in our DNA, which is like the instruction manual for our body. It helps make sure everything is working properly and the right things are turned on and off at the right times.

Unfortunately, as we get older, our body doesn't make as much NAD+ as it used to, and this can cause problems.

Benefits of NAD+:

NAD+ is known for its many benefits in the body, including improved energy metabolism, increased mitochondrial function, reduced inflammation, and improved cognitive function. It has also been shown to have neuroprotective effects, improve athletic performance, and support detoxification pathways in the body.

Dosage recommendations

The recommended dosage of NAD+ for IV administration can vary depending on the individual's needs and the specific health condition being treated. In general, IV doses of NAD+ are administered under the supervision of a healthcare professional and can range from 250 mg to 1000 mg per infusion. The frequency and duration of NAD+ infusions can also vary depending on the individual's needs and response to treatment.

Conditions treated with NAD+

NAD+ infusion therapy has been used to treat a variety of health conditions, including addiction, chronic fatigue syndrome, fibromyalgia, neurodegenerative disorders, and mitochondrial disorders. It has also been used as a complementary therapy for cancer patients undergoing chemotherapy.

Signs of NAD+ deficiency

Signs of NAD+ deficiency can include fatigue, brain fog, decreased physical and mental performance, decreased immune function, and a higher risk of chronic diseases.

Signs of NAD+ toxicity

Signs of NAD+ toxicity are rare, but can include flushing, dizziness, nausea, and headache.

Contraindications

NAD+ infusion therapy may not be suitable for individuals with a history of severe liver or kidney disease, or certain genetic disorders. It is also contraindicated for pregnant or breastfeeding women.

Who is a good candidate to receive NAD+ infusion

Individuals who are seeking support for energy metabolism, cognitive function, and overall health may benefit from NAD+ infusion therapy. It may also be suitable for individuals with certain health conditions, such as addiction, chronic fatigue syndrome, or neurodegenerative disorders.

Is NAD+ used with other compounds

Glutathione can be combined with NAD+ in an infusion. In fact, the combination of NAD+ and glutathione in an IV infusion has been used to treat various health conditions, including Parkinson's disease, chronic fatigue syndrome, and fibromyalgia.

Glutathione is a powerful antioxidant that helps to protect cells from oxidative stress and damage. It plays a critical role in many cellular processes, including detoxification, immune function, and energy metabolism. When combined with NAD+, glutathione may help to support cellular function and improve overall health.

The combination of NAD+ and glutathione in an IV infusion may be particularly beneficial for individuals who are seeking support for energy metabolism, cognitive function, and detoxification pathways.

It is important to note that glutathione should be administered separately after the infusion. Do not put glutathione in the NAD infusion.

Frequency of treatments

The frequency of NAD+ infusion therapy can vary depending on the individual's needs and response to treatment. Some individuals may benefit from weekly or bi-weekly infusions, while others may require infusions less frequently.

One anecdotal recommendation is 10gm IV in 4 months. Please note that there are no guidelines for optimal doses of NAD+ or frequency and this should be based on patient needs and discussed with your medical director.

Special Notes

NAD+ can be light-sensitive, especially when in solution. Exposure to light can cause NAD+ to degrade and lose its biological activity.

Therefore, it is important to protect NAD+ from light during storage and handling.

To prevent light-induced degradation, NAD+ should be stored in a dark container or wrapped in aluminum foil to protect it from light exposure. Additionally, it is recommended to use freshly prepared NAD+ solutions for IV infusion to ensure maximal potency and efficacy.

NAD+ is sensitive to oxygen and can be rapidly degraded in the presence of oxygen. This is because NAD+ contains a highly oxidizable nicotinamide ring, which can undergo oxidative damage in the presence of oxygen. To minimize oxidative damage to NAD+, it is typically prepared and stored in an oxygen-free environment, such as a nitrogen or argon atmosphere, and handled with care to avoid exposure to air. Precautions should be taken not to inject any air into the vial when removing NAD+.

Symptoms occur in most cases of NAD+ administration such as epigastric pressure, head wooziness, heavy arms, etc. and are related to speed at which the drip is flowing.. Slow the drip down for immediate resolution, and then titrate back up as tolerated. Do not encourage the patient to "push through" the symptoms. Let the patient know these will occur and that the symptoms will pass. Titrating has an immediate response.

Overall, NAD+ infusion therapy has shown promising results in improving energy metabolism, cognitive function, and overall health. Further research is needed to determine the optimal dosages, duration, and frequency of NAD+ infusion therapy for different health conditions.

Clinical Information

1. What forms does NAD+ come in?

   NAD+ supplements are available in various forms, including capsules, tablets, and IV formulations.

2. What are the daily dosage limits?

   There is no established daily dosage limit for NAD+ supplements, as the optimal dosage and duration of supplementation may vary depending on the individual's needs and response to treatment.

3. How is NAD+ stored?

   NAD+ supplements should be stored in a cool, dry place, away from direct sunlight and heat.

4. How is NAD+ prepared for IV infusion?

   NAD+ can be prepared for IV infusion by reconstituting it with sterile water or saline solution. The prepared solution should be used immediately or refrigerated for later use. It is important to use freshly prepared NAD+ solutions for IV infusion to ensure maximal potency and efficacy.

5. Treatment protocols:

   NAD+ has been studied for its potential therapeutic benefits in various health conditions, including neurodegenerative diseases, addiction, and chronic fatigue syndrome. However, the optimal dosage and duration of NAD+ supplementation for different health conditions have not been fully established and may vary depending on the individual's needs and response to treatment. For example, for the treatment of addiction, a standard protocol may involve daily IV infusions of NAD+ for up to 10 days. For the treatment of chronic fatigue syndrome, a protocol may involve weekly IV infusions of NAD+ for up to 12 weeks.

6. What is the half-life of NAD+?
    The half-life of NAD+ in the body is relatively short, with a half-life of approximately 15 minutes. This short half-life means that NAD+ levels can decline rapidly under conditions of high oxidative stress or toxin exposure.

7. Is it stable?
    NAD+ is a relatively unstable compound that is affected by heat, light, and air.

References

1. Belenky P, Bogan KL, Brenner C. NAD+ metabolism in health and disease. Trends in biochemical sciences. 2007 Aug 31;32(1):12-9.

2. Henning RJ. NAD+ and NADH in Cellular Functions and Disease: Relevance to Aging and Aging-Related Disease. Oxidative Medicine and Cellular Longevity. 2018 Oct 15;2018.

3. Kennedy DO. B vitamins and the brain: mechanisms, dose and efficacy--a review. Nutrients. 2016 Feb;8(2):68.

5. IV infusion of reduced glutathione and nicotinamide adenine dinucleotide (NADH) in treatment of Parkinson's disease. Pharmacology, biochemistry, and behavior. 1990 Oct 1;35(2):453-4.

6. Birkmayer JG, Vrecko C, Volc D, Birkmayer W. Nicotinamide adenine dinucleotide (NADH)--a new therapeutic approach to Parkinson's disease. Comparison of oral and parenteral application. Acta Neurologica Scandinavica. 1993 Jul;146(Suppl):32-5.

Lipoic Acid

Lipoic acid and alpha-lipoic acid (ALA) are two terms that are often used interchangeably to refer to the same compound. Alpha-lipoic acid is actually the biologically active form of lipoic acid and is the form that is most commonly used in dietary supplements and IV infusions.

ALA is considered a coenzyme involved in the breakdown of glucose to produce energy and is also involved in the synthesis of ATP, the primary energy source for cells. ALA is also a potent antioxidant and helps to neutralize free radicals, which can cause oxidative damage to cells and contribute to various diseases.

ALA is not considered an essential nutrient because the body can produce it on its own. However, supplementation with ALA has been shown to provide various health benefits, particularly in the areas of metabolic health and oxidative stress.

Benefits of alpha lipoic acid:

ALA has been shown to have numerous benefits in the body, including improved glucose metabolism, enhanced insulin sensitivity, reduced inflammation, and improved antioxidant defense. ALA may also have neuroprotective effects and has been studied for its potential therapeutic benefits in various neurological disorders.

Dosage recommendations

The recommended dosage of ALA for IV administration can vary depending on the individual's needs and the specific health condition being treated. In general, IV doses of ALA range from 300 to 600 mg per infusion. The frequency and duration of ALA infusions can also vary depending on the individual's needs and response to treatment.

Conditions treated with alpha lipoic acid

ALA infusion therapy has been used to treat a variety of health conditions, including diabetic neuropathy, metabolic syndrome, hepatitis C, and neurodegenerative disorders such as Alzheimer's and Parkinson's disease. ALA has also been studied for its potential therapeutic benefits in cardiovascular disease and cancer.

Signs of alpha lipoic acid deficiency

There are no specific signs of ALA deficiency, as the body can synthesize it on its own. However, individuals with certain health conditions, such as liver disease or diabetes, may have lower levels of ALA in the body.

Signs of alpha lipoic acid toxicity

Signs of ALA toxicity are rare, but can include gastrointestinal disturbances, skin rash, and hypoglycemia in individuals with diabetes.

In rare cases, IV ALA infusion therapy has been associated with anaphylactic reactions, a severe and potentially life-threatening allergic reaction. Signs of anaphylaxis may include difficulty breathing, swelling of the face or throat, rapid heart rate, and decreased blood pressure.

Contraindications

ALA infusion therapy may not be suitable for individuals with a history of thiamine deficiency, as it can interfere with thiamine absorption. It is also contraindicated for pregnant or breastfeeding women.

Who is a good candidate to receive alpha lipoic acid infusion

Individuals who are seeking support for metabolic health, oxidative stress, and neurological function may benefit from ALA infusion therapy. It may also be suitable for individuals with certain health conditions, such as diabetic neuropathy or neurodegenerative disorders.

Is alpha lipoic acid used with other compounds:

ALA infusion therapy is often combined with other compounds, such as amino acids, vitamins, and minerals, to support overall health and wellness. Some of these compounds may include magnesium, vitamin B complex, vitamin C, and glutathione.

Frequency of treatments

The frequency of ALA infusion therapy can vary depending on the individual's needs and response to treatment. Some individuals may benefit from weekly or bi-weekly infusions, while others may require infusions less frequently.

Clinical Information

1. What forms does alpha lipoic acid come in?

   Alpha lipoic acid is a natural compound that is found in small amounts in certain foods, such as spinach, broccoli, and organ meats. Alpha lipoic acid supplements are also available in various forms, including capsules, tablets, and IV formulations.

2. What are the daily dosage limits?

   The optimal dosage of alpha lipoic acid may vary depending on the individual's needs and response to treatment. However, the generally recommended daily dosage of alpha lipoic acid supplements is 200-600 milligrams, taken in divided doses throughout the day. Higher doses of alpha lipoic acid may be used under the guidance of a healthcare professional.

3. How is alpha lipoic acid stored?

   Alpha lipoic acid supplements should be stored in a cool, dry place, away from direct sunlight and heat.

4. How is alpha lipoic acid prepared for IV infusion?

   Alpha lipoic acid can be prepared for IV infusion by reconstituting it with sterile water or saline solution. The prepared solution should be used immediately or refrigerated for later use. It is important to use freshly prepared alpha lipoic acid solutions for IV infusion to ensure maximal potency and efficacy.

5. Treatment protocols:

Alpha lipoic acid has been studied for its potential therapeutic benefits in various health conditions, including diabetic neuropathy, antioxidant support, and liver disease. However, the optimal dosage and duration of alpha lipoic acid supplementation for different health conditions have not been fully established and may vary depending on the individual's needs and response to treatment. For example, for the treatment of diabetic neuropathy, a standard protocol may involve daily doses of 600 milligrams of alpha lipoic acid for up to 3 weeks. For the treatment of liver disease, a protocol may involve weekly IV infusions of 600 milligrams of alpha lipoic acid for up to 12 weeks.

6. What is the half-life of alpha lipoic acid?

The half-life of alpha lipoic acid in the body is relatively short, with a half-life of approximately 30 minutes. This short half-life means that alpha lipoic acid levels can decline rapidly under conditions of high oxidative stress or toxin exposure.

7. Is it stable?

Alpha lipoic acid is a relatively stable compound that is not affected by heat, light, or air. However, alpha lipoic acid supplements should be stored in a cool, dry place, away from direct sunlight and heat, to ensure maximal potency and efficacy.

References

1. Packer L, Witt EH, Tritschler HJ. Alpha-lipoic acid as a biological antioxidant. Free radical biology and medicine. 1995 Aug 1;19(2):227-50.

2. Suh JH, Shenvi SV, Dixon BM, Liu H, Jaiswal AK, Liu RM, Hagen TM. Decline in transcriptional activity of Nrf2 causes age-related loss of glutathione synthesis, which is reversible with lipoic acid. Proceedings of the National Academy of Sciences. 2004 Mar 2;101(10):3381-6.

3. Zembron-Lacny A, Gajewski M, Naczk M, Siatkowski I. Effect of alpha-lipoic acid supplementation on plasma adiponectin, cystatin C and kidney function in cardiac surgery patients. Annals of clinical biochemistry. 2016 Sep;53(5):570-7.

4. Ziegler D, Hanefeld M, Ruhnau KJ, Hasche H, Lobisch M, Schütte K, Kerum G, Malessa R. Treatment of symptomatic diabetic peripheral neuropathy with the antioxidant alpha-lipoic acid: a 3-week multicentre randomized controlled trial (ALADIN Study). Diabetologia. 1995 Dec 1;38(12):1425-33.

5. Biewenga GP, Haenen GR, Bast A. The pharmacology of the antioxidant lipoic acid. General pharmacology. 1997 Mar 1;29(3):315-31.

CHAPTER 7 - ESSENTIAL NUTRIENT LIKE COMPOUNDS

CHOLINE

Choline is an essential nutrient that plays a crucial role in various physiological processes, including cell membrane integrity, neurotransmitter synthesis, fat metabolism, and maintenance of liver function. It is a precursor to the neurotransmitter acetylcholine, which is involved in memory, muscle control, and mood regulation.

Benefits of Choline

Some of the benefits of choline include:

1. Cognitive function support: Choline has been shown to enhance memory and learning abilities, making it an essential nutrient for maintaining cognitive health.

2. Liver health: Choline plays a role in fat metabolism, helping to prevent the accumulation of fat in the liver and reducing the risk of fatty liver disease.

3. Cardiovascular health: Choline has been suggested to reduce homocysteine levels, which may contribute to a decreased risk of cardiovascular diseases.

4. Nervous system support: Choline is essential for the synthesis of neurotransmitters, which play a vital role in maintaining healthy nerve function.

Dosage Recommendations

The appropriate dosage of choline in IV hydration therapy depends on the individual's age, sex, medical history, and overall health. Healthcare professionals should determine the specific dosage based on the patient's needs and the goals of treatment. The Adequate Intake (AI) for choline for adults is 425 mg/day for women and 550 mg/day for men. However, the therapeutic dosage in IV hydration may vary and should be determined by a healthcare professional.

Conditions Treated with Choline

Some conditions that may benefit from choline supplementation in IV hydration therapy include:

1. Cognitive decline or memory impairment

2. Fatty liver disease

3. Depression and anxiety

4. Neurological disorders

5. High homocysteine levels

Signs of Choline Deficiency

Choline deficiency is rare but can occur in certain situations, such as strict vegetarian diets or specific genetic mutations. Signs of choline deficiency may include fatigue, memory problems, muscle aches, mood disturbances, or liver dysfunction

Signs of Choline Toxicity

Excessive choline intake can lead to choline toxicity, which may present as nausea, vomiting, diarrhea, hypotension, fishy body odor, or increased salivation.

Contraindications

Choline supplementation in IV hydration therapy may be contraindicated in individuals with certain medical conditions or taking specific medications. Individuals with trimethylaminuria (TMAU), also known as fish odor syndrome. Choline can exacerbate the symptoms of this condition, as it is metabolized into trimethylamine, which has a fishy odor. People with bipolar disorder or a history of mania. Choline is a precursor to the neurotransmitter acetylcholine, and high levels of acetylcholine have been associated with manic episodes in some individuals with bipolar disorder. Individuals with kidney or liver disease may need to be cautious with choline supplementation, as the metabolism and excretion of choline can be affected by impaired kidney or liver function. In such cases, a healthcare professional should carefully monitor choline intake. People taking medications that interact with choline, such as anticholinergic drugs, which block the effects of acetylcholine. Choline supplementation may interfere with the effectiveness of these medications.

Who is a Good Candidate to Receive Choline Infusion

Individuals with choline deficiency, cognitive decline, liver dysfunction, or high homocysteine levels may be good candidates for choline IV therapy. However, a healthcare professional should assess each patient's unique needs and medical history to determine if choline infusion is appropriate.

Is Choline Used with Other Compounds

Choline is often combined with other vitamins, minerals, and nutrients in IV hydration therapy to enhance its effects and provide comprehensive support. For example, it may be included in a "Myers' Cocktail" or other nutrient infusion formulas.

Frequency of Treatments

The frequency of choline IV treatments will depend on the patient's specific needs, the severity of the deficiency or condition being treated, and the healthcare provider's recommendations. Treatment frequency may range from weekly to monthly, depending on the individual case.

Special Notes

Choline is a component of a popular weight loss infusion known as the "MIC" (Methionine,

Inositol, and Choline) cocktail. This combination is believed to help boost metabolism, support liver function, and promote fat breakdown, thereby aiding in weight loss efforts. However, it is essential to note that choline supplementation should be used in conjunction with a balanced diet and regular exercise to achieve optimal weight loss results.

The MIC (Methionine, Inositol, and Choline) cocktail is administered as an intramuscular (IM) injection rather than intravenous (IV) infusion. These injections are typically given in a series as part of a weight loss program or to support liver function. The frequency of MIC injections may vary depending on the individual's specific needs, but they are often administered on a weekly basis.

Clinical Information

1. What forms does choline come in?
   Choline is an essential nutrient that is available in supplement form, such as capsules and tablets. It is also present in small amounts in certain foods, such as eggs, liver, and peanuts.

2. What are the daily dosage limits?
   The recommended daily intake of choline varies by age, gender, and health status. For adults, the recommended daily intake of choline is 425-550 milligrams per day. It is important to not exceed the tolerable upper intake level (UL) of choline, which is set at 3500 milligrams per day for adults.

3. How is choline stored?
   Choline supplements should be stored in a cool, dry place, away from direct sunlight and heat.

4. How is choline prepared for IV infusion?
   Choline can be prepared for IV infusion by diluting it in sterile water or saline solution. The prepared solution should be used immediately or refrigerated for later use. It is

important to use freshly prepared choline solutions for IV infusion to ensure maximal potency and efficacy.

5. Treatment protocols:
    Choline supplementation has been studied for its potential therapeutic benefits in various health conditions, such as liver disease and cognitive function. However, the optimal dosage and duration of choline supplementation for different health conditions have not been fully established and may vary depending on the individual's needs and response to treatment.

6. What is the half-life of choline?
    The half-life of choline in the body varies depending on the form of choline and individual metabolism, with an average half-life of around 1-2 hours.

7. Is it stable?
    Choline is a relatively stable compound that is not affected by heat or light. It can be degraded by exposure to air and moisture, so choline supplements should be stored in a cool, dry place, away from direct sunlight and heat, to ensure maximal potency and efficacy.

References

1. Zeisel, S. H., & da Costa, K. A. (2009). Choline: an essential nutrient for public health. Nutrition reviews, 67(11), 615-623.

2. Poly, C., Massaro, J. M., Seshadri, S., Wolf, P. A., Cho, E., Krall, E., ... & Au, R. (2011). The relation of dietary choline

to cognitive performance and white-matter hyperintensity in the Framingham Offspring Cohort. The American journal of clinical nutrition, 94(6), 1584-1591.

3. Ueland, P. M., Holm, P. I., & Hustad, S. (2005). Betaine: a key modulator of one-carbon metabolism and homocysteine status. Clinical chemistry and laboratory medicine, 43(10), 1069-1075.

4. Corbin, K. D., & Zeisel, S. H. (2012). Choline metabolism provides novel insights into nonalcoholic fatty liver disease and its progression. Current opinion in gastroenterology, 28(2), 159-165.

5. Gao, X., Randell, E., Zhou, H., & Sun, G. (2016). Higher serum choline and betaine levels are associated with better body composition in male but not female population. PLoS One, 11(3), e0150762.

INOSITOL

Inositol, sometimes referred to as myo-inositol, is a naturally occurring sugar alcohol found in various foods, including fruits, beans, grains, and nuts. It plays a crucial role in cellular signaling and is involved in various physiological processes such as insulin sensitivity, neurotransmitter modulation, and lipid metabolism.

Benefits of Inositol

Some of the main benefits of inositol include:

1. Mood regulation: Inositol has been shown to positively influence serotonin and dopamine receptors, which may help improve mood and reduce symptoms of anxiety and depression.

2. Insulin sensitivity: Inositol has been linked to improved insulin sensitivity, potentially benefiting individuals with insulin resistance or type 2 diabetes.

3. Polycystic ovary syndrome (PCOS) management: Studies suggest that inositol supplementation may help improve hormonal balance and metabolic markers in women with PCOS.

4. Fertility: Inositol may enhance ovarian function and support healthy egg development, potentially benefiting fertility in women with PCOS.

5. Lipid metabolism: Inositol has been associated with improved lipid metabolism, which can help maintain healthy cholesterol levels and support liver function.

Dosage Recommendations

The appropriate dosage of inositol in IV hydration therapy depends on factors such as the individual's age, sex, medical history, and overall health. While there is no established recommended daily intake for inositol, oral supplementation doses typically range from 500 mg to 18 g per day, depending on the condition being treated. The therapeutic dosage for IV inositol may vary, and healthcare professionals should determine the specific dosage based on the patient's needs and treatment goals.

Conditions Treated with Inositol

Some conditions that may benefit from inositol supplementation in IV hydration therapy include:

1. Mood disorders, such as depression and anxiety

2. Insulin resistance or type 2 diabetes

3. Polycystic ovary syndrome (PCOS)

4. Fertility issues related to PCOS

5. High cholesterol levels or fatty liver disease

Signs of Inositol Deficiency

Inositol deficiency is rare, as the body can produce it in small amounts and obtain it through dietary sources. However, certain situations, such as poor diet or specific medical conditions, may lead to a deficiency. Signs of inositol deficiency may include mood disturbances such as anxiety or depression, insulin resistance, polycystic ovary syndrome (PCOS) symptoms, and fertility issues.

Signs of Inositol Toxicity

Inositol toxicity is uncommon, but excessive intake may cause some side effects, such as gastrointestinal issues, including nausea, gas, or diarrhea, dizziness or fatigue.

Contraindications

Inositol supplementation in IV hydration therapy may be contraindicated in individuals with certain medical conditions or taking specific medications. Antidepressants: Inositol may affect the serotonin system in the brain, which is also targeted by certain antidepressant medications, such as selective serotonin reuptake inhibitors (SSRIs). While there is no definitive evidence of an interaction, caution is advised when combining inositol with these medications.

1. Lithium: Inositol may reduce the effectiveness of lithium, a medication used to treat bipolar disorder. This is because lithium works by decreasing inositol levels in the brain, and taking inositol supplements could counteract this effect.

2. Antipsychotic medications: Some antipsychotic medications, such as olanzapine and clozapine, may also affect inositol levels in the brain. While there is limited evidence of an interaction, it is essential to exercise caution and consult a healthcare provider when considering inositol supplementation while taking these medications.

3. Anti-anxiety medications: Inositol has been studied for its potential benefits in reducing anxiety symptoms. While it is not clear if there are direct interactions, combining inositol with anti-anxiety medications may enhance their effects, potentially leading to excessive sedation or other side effects. Consult your healthcare provider before combining inositol with anti-anxiety medications.

Who is a Good Candidate to Receive Inositol Infusion

Individuals with mood disorders, insulin resistance, PCOS, fertility issues, or lipid metabolism problems may be good candidates for inositol IV therapy. However, a healthcare professional should assess each patient's unique needs and medical history to determine if inositol infusion is appropriate.

Is Inositol Used with Other Compounds

Inositol is often combined with other vitamins, minerals, and nutrients in IV hydration therapy to enhance its effects and provide comprehensive support. For example, it may be included in a "Myers' Cocktail" or other nutrient infusion formulas. It is more common to ingest inositol as oral supplementation.

Frequency of Treatments

The frequency of inositol IV treatments will depend on the patient's specific needs, the severity of the deficiency or condition being treated, and the healthcare provider's recommendations. Treatment frequency may range from weekly to monthly, depending on the individual case.

Special Notes

Inositol is a component of a popular weight loss infusion known as the "MIC" (Methionine, Inositol, and Choline) cocktail. This combination is believed to help boost metabolism, support liver function, and promote fat breakdown, thereby aiding in weight loss efforts. However, it is essential to note that inositol supplementation should be used in conjunction with a balanced diet and regular exercise to achieve optimal weight loss results.

Clinical Information

1. What forms does inositol come in?
   Inositol is available in various forms, including capsules, tablets, powders, and IV formulations.

2. What are the daily dosage limits?
   The optimal dosage of inositol may vary depending on the individual's needs and response to treatment. However, the generally recommended daily dosage of inositol supplements ranges from 500 to 4000 milligrams, taken in divided doses throughout the day.

3. How is inositol stored?
   Inositol supplements should be stored in a cool, dry place, away from direct sunlight and heat.

4. How is inositol prepared for IV infusion?
   Inositol can be prepared for IV infusion by dissolving it in sterile water or saline solution. The prepared solution should be used immediately or refrigerated for later use. It is important to use freshly prepared inositol solutions for IV infusion to ensure maximal potency and efficacy.

5. Treatment protocols:
   Inositol has been studied for its potential therapeutic benefits in various health conditions, including anxiety, depression,

and polycystic ovary syndrome (PCOS). However, the optimal dosage and duration of inositol supplementation for different health conditions have not been fully established and may vary depending on the individual's needs and response to treatment. For example, for the treatment of anxiety and depression, a standard protocol may involve daily doses of 12-18 grams of inositol for up to 6 weeks. For the treatment of PCOS, a protocol may involve daily doses of 2-4 grams of inositol for up to 3 months.

6. What is the half-life of inositol?

The half-life of inositol in the body is relatively short, with a half-life of approximately 4 hours. This short half-life means that inositol levels can rapidly decrease after supplementation is discontinued.

7. Is it stable?

Inositol is a relatively stable compound that is not affected by heat or light. It is highly soluble in water and is not easily degraded by enzymes in the body. However, inositol supplements should be stored properly to ensure maximal potency and efficacy.

References

1. Levine, J. (1997). Controlled trials of inositol in psychiatry. European Neuropsychopharmacology, 7(2), 147-155.

2. Genazzani, A. D., Lanzoni, C., Ricchieri, F., & Jasonni, V. M. (2008). Myo-inositol administration positively affects

hyperinsulinemia and hormonal parameters in overweight patients with polycystic ovary syndrome. Gynecological Endocrinology, 24(3), 139-144.

3. Unfer, V., Carlomagno, G., Dante, G., & Facchinetti, F. (2012). Effects of myo-inositol in women with PCOS: a systematic review of randomized controlled trials. Gynecological Endocrinology, 28(7), 509-515.

4. Dinicola, S., Minini, M., Unfer, V., Verna, R., Cucina, A., & Bizzarri, M. (2017). Nutritional and acquired deficiencies in inositol bioavailability. Correlations with metabolic disorders. International Journal of Molecular Sciences, 18(10), 2187.

NUTRIENT LIKE COMPOUNDS

There are several other compounds that are not used in IV therapy, but are considered essential nutrients, and are important for overall health and well-being. Being knowledgeable about these compounds can supplement IV therapy in between sessions. These include:

Phytochemicals:

These are naturally occurring compounds found in plants, such as carotenoids, flavonoids, and resveratrol. They have antioxidant and anti-inflammatory properties, and may help protect against chronic diseases like cancer and heart disease.

The best sources of phytochemicals are a diverse range of whole, unprocessed plant-based foods, including fruits, vegetables, whole grains, legumes, nuts, seeds, herbs, and spices.

Some examples of phytochemical-rich food sources include:

1. Berries (e.g., blueberries, strawberries, raspberries, blackberries) - rich in anthocyanins and flavonoids

2. Cruciferous vegetables (e.g., broccoli, cauliflower, kale, Brussels sprouts) - contain sulforaphane, indoles, and isothiocyanates

3. Tomatoes - a good source of lycopene

4. Leafy greens (e.g., spinach, collard greens, Swiss chard) - high in carotenoids, lutein, and zeaxanthin

5. Grapes and red wine - rich in resveratrol and other polyphenols

6. Citrus fruits (e.g., oranges, lemons, grapefruits) - contain flavonoids, such as hesperidin and naringenin

7. Green tea - a good source of catechins, particularly epigallocatechin-3-gallate (EGCG)

8. Dark chocolate and cocoa - high in flavanols and other polyphenols

9. Legumes (e.g., beans, lentils, chickpeas) - contain various phytochemicals, such as isoflavones, phytic acid, and saponins

10. Nuts and seeds (e.g., walnuts, flaxseeds, chia seeds) - rich in lignans and other phytochemicals

11. Herbs and spices (e.g., turmeric, ginger, cinnamon, rosemary) - contain a wide variety of phytochemicals, including curcumin, gingerol, and cinnamaldehyde

To maximize the health benefits of phytochemicals, it is recommended to consume a diverse and colorful array of plant-based foods, as different colors and food types offer various phytochemicals with distinct health-promoting properties. Incorporating a wide range of fruits, vegetables, whole grains, legumes, nuts, seeds, herbs, and spices into your diet can help ensure an adequate intake of these beneficial compounds.

Fiber

Although not technically a nutrient, fiber is a type of carbohydrate that the body cannot digest. It helps regulate digestion and bowel movements, and may also lower cholesterol and blood sugar levels.

The best sources of fiber are plant-based foods, including whole grains, fruits, vegetables, legumes, nuts, and seeds. Here are some excellent sources of dietary fiber:

1. Whole grains: Whole wheat, brown rice, quinoa, barley, oats, and bulgur are rich in fiber. Opt for whole-grain bread, pasta, and cereals to increase your fiber intake.

2. Fruits: Raspberries, blackberries, pears, apples (with the skin), oranges, and bananas are good sources of fiber. Eating a variety of fruits ensures a balanced intake of both soluble and insoluble fibers.

3. Vegetables: Leafy greens, broccoli, cauliflower, Brussels sprouts, sweet potatoes, carrots, and artichokes are fiber-rich choices. Including a variety of vegetables in your diet can help increase your overall fiber intake.

4. Legumes: Beans (e.g., black beans, kidney beans, pinto beans, white beans), lentils, and chickpeas are excellent sources of fiber. They can be added to salads, soups, stews, and other dishes for a fiber boost.

5. Nuts and seeds: Almonds, pistachios, chia seeds, flaxseeds, and sunflower seeds are all high in fiber. Incorporate them into your diet as snacks, in salads, or as toppings for yogurt or oatmeal.

6. Psyllium husk: This natural dietary fiber supplement is derived from the seed husks of the Plantago ovata plant. It can be added to smoothies, oatmeal, or yogurt to increase fiber intake.

Probiotics

Probiotics are live microorganisms, primarily bacteria and yeasts, that provide various health benefits when consumed in adequate amounts. They help maintain a healthy balance of gut bacteria, support digestion, and enhance immune function. The best sources of probiotics are fermented foods, as the fermentation process encourages the growth of beneficial microorganisms. Some excellent sources of probiotics include:

1. Yogurt: One of the most popular probiotic foods, yogurt is made by fermenting milk with specific bacteria, such as Lactobacillus and Bifidobacterium strains. Look for yogurt with "live and active cultures" on the label, which indicates the presence of probiotics.

2. Kefir: This fermented milk drink is similar to yogurt but has a thinner consistency and is made by fermenting milk with a mixture of bacteria and yeasts, known as kefir grains. Kefir often contains a broader range of probiotics than yogurt.

3. Sauerkraut: Made from fermented cabbage, sauerkraut is rich in probiotics, particularly Lactobacillus strains. Ensure that the sauerkraut you choose is unpasteurized, as the pasteurization process can kill the beneficial bacteria.

4. Kimchi: This traditional Korean dish is made from fermented vegetables, primarily cabbage, and is seasoned with various spices. Kimchi is a rich source of probiotics, including Lactobacillus and other beneficial bacteria.

5. Tempeh: This fermented soybean product is a popular plant-based protein source and is rich in probiotics, particularly the Rhizopus oligosporus strain.

6. Miso: A traditional Japanese seasoning made from fermented soybeans, miso is a rich source of probiotics, including Lactobacillus and Bifidobacterium strains. It is commonly used in soups and sauces.

7. Kombucha: This fermented tea beverage contains a mixture of bacteria and yeasts that provide probiotic benefits. Kombucha can be found in various flavors and is becoming increasingly popular as a probiotic drink.

8. Pickles: Fermented pickles made in a saltwater brine are a good source of Lactobacillus bacteria. Note that pickles made with vinegar do not contain live probiotics.

9. Traditional buttermilk: Traditional buttermilk, which is the liquid remaining after churning butter, is a source of probiotics. However, most commercially available buttermilk is cultured, meaning it is made by adding bacteria to milk, and may not have the same probiotic benefits as traditional buttermilk.

Including a variety of these fermented foods in your diet can help ensure a diverse and adequate intake of probiotics to support gut health. In addition to these food sources, probiotic supplements are also available, but it is essential to consult a healthcare provider before starting any supplementation.

Prebiotics

Prebiotics are non-digestible fibers that serve as food for probiotics, the beneficial bacteria in your gut. They help promote the growth and activity of probiotics, which in turn support digestive health and overall well-being. The best sources of prebiotics are plant-based foods rich in specific types of fibers, such as inulin, oligofructose, and galacto-oligosaccharides (GOS). Some excellent sources of prebiotic-rich foods include:

1. Chicory root: One of the richest sources of inulin, a prebiotic fiber, chicory root can be used as a coffee substitute or added to various recipes to increase fiber intake.

2. Jerusalem artichoke: Also known as the sunchoke, Jerusalem artichokes are tubers that are high in inulin and can be consumed raw, cooked, or roasted.

3. Dandelion greens: These leafy greens are rich in prebiotic fibers and can be added to salads, soups, or sautéed as a side dish.

4. Garlic: Garlic contains inulin and other prebiotic fibers, making it a flavorful addition to many recipes while also promoting gut health.

5. Onions: Both raw and cooked onions are a good source of prebiotic fibers, such as inulin and oligofructose.

6. Leeks: Leeks, which are part of the onion family, are also rich in prebiotic fibers and can be added to soups, stews, and other dishes.

7. Asparagus: This versatile vegetable is a good source of inulin and can be prepared in various ways, including steaming, grilling, or roasting.

8. Bananas: While all bananas contain some prebiotic fibers, unripe (green) bananas are particularly rich in resistant starch, which serves as a prebiotic.

9. Whole grains: Whole grains, such as barley, oats, and whole wheat, contain prebiotic fibers like beta-glucan and oligosaccharides, which promote the growth of beneficial gut bacteria.

10. Legumes: Beans, lentils, and chickpeas are rich in prebiotic fibers and resistant starch, making them an excellent addition to a gut-friendly diet.

Including a variety of these prebiotic-rich foods in your diet can help support the growth and activity of beneficial gut bacteria and promote overall digestive health. Combining prebiotic-rich foods with probiotic-rich foods or supplements can create a synergistic effect, enhancing the benefits of both for optimal gut health.

Omega-3 Fatty Acids

These are a type of polyunsaturated fat that is important for brain and heart health. They may also have anti-inflammatory properties and help reduce the risk of chronic diseases. Omega-3 fatty acids, specifically eicosapentaenoic acid (EPA), docosahexaenoic acid (DHA), and alpha-linolenic acid (ALA), are essential nutrients that play crucial roles in maintaining heart health, brain function, and reducing inflammation in the body. The best sources of omega-3 fatty acids vary depending on the specific type:

1. Fatty fish: The most abundant sources of EPA and DHA are fatty fish, such as salmon, mackerel, sardines, anchovies, herring, and trout. It is recommended to consume at least two servings of fatty fish per week to ensure adequate intake of EPA and DHA.

2. Fish oil: Fish oil supplements derived from fish like cod, salmon, or krill are another rich source of EPA and DHA. They can be a good option for individuals who do not consume fish regularly or have difficulty meeting their omega-3 needs through diet alone.

3. Algae oil: Microalgae are the primary producers of DHA in the marine food chain. Algae oil supplements are a suitable option for vegans and vegetarians who want to obtain DHA without consuming fish or fish oil.

4. Chia seeds: These nutrient-dense seeds are an excellent plant-based source of ALA, a precursor to EPA and DHA. Other seeds like flaxseeds and hemp seeds are also high in ALA.

5. Walnuts: Among nuts, walnuts contain the highest amount of ALA, making them a valuable source of plant-based omega-3 fatty acids.

6. Plant oils: Certain plant oils, such as flaxseed oil, canola oil, and soybean oil, are rich sources of ALA.

It is important to note that the conversion of ALA to EPA and DHA in the human body is inefficient, which means that consuming plant-based sources of omega-3s may not provide the same benefits as those from fatty fish. However, including a variety of plant-based sources of ALA can still contribute to overall omega-3 intake and provide health benefits, especially for vegetarians and vegans.

To ensure an adequate intake of omega-3 fatty acids, aim to include a combination of fatty fish, plant-based sources of ALA, or high-quality supplements in your diet.

CHAPTER 8 - PEPTIDES

*Disclaimer - There are regulations governing the use of peptides in medicine and research. In the United States, the Food and Drug Administration (FDA) regulates the use of peptides as drugs. Peptides that are used in research are also subject to regulations set by organizations such as the National Institutes of Health (NIH) and the International Council for Harmonisation of Technical Requirements for Pharmaceuticals for Human Use (ICH). These regulatory bodies set standards for the safety and efficacy of peptides and monitor their use in clinical trials and approved medical treatments.

It is important to note that the use of peptides for non-medical purposes, such as in sports performance enhancement or cosmetic treatments, may not be regulated in the same way and may carry additional risks. The information in this chapter is for educational purposes only. Any protocols you create must be approved by your medical director and should be for the benefit of your clients.

Peptides are short chains of amino acids that can have various biological functions in the body. While amino acids are the building blocks of proteins, peptides have unique structures and functions that can be beneficial for health and wellness. This unique structure allows peptides to be easily absorbed and utilized by the body due to their small size and specific sequences of amino acids.

This structure also allows peptides to be more stable than free amino acids, which can break down easily in the body. Additionally, peptides can be designed to target specific biological processes and functions in the body, making them potentially more effective than amino acids in delivering specific health benefits. Overall, these unique structural features of peptides make them beneficial for health and wellness purposes.

Here are some reasons why peptides may be used instead of amino acids for health and wellness:

1. Specificity: Peptides can be designed to target specific biological processes and functions in the body. For example, certain peptides can stimulate the production of collagen, which can improve skin health and reduce wrinkles.

2. Bioavailability: Peptides can be easily absorbed and utilized by the body due to their small size and structure. This means that they can be more effective than amino acids when it comes to delivering specific health benefits.

3. Stability: Peptides are more stable than free amino acids, which can break down easily in the body. This means that peptides can be more effective in delivering their intended health benefits over time.

4. Safety: Peptides are generally safe for human consumption, as they are naturally occurring compounds in the body. However, as with any supplement, it's important to consult

with a healthcare professional before using peptides for health and wellness purposes.

Overall, peptides offer a unique and effective approach to supporting various aspects of health and wellness.

Some peptides have been studied for their effects on muscle growth, weight loss, anti-aging, and overall health though more research is needed to fully understand their efficacy and safety. Some of the most commonly used peptides in health and wellness include:

1. BPC-157: BPC stands for "Body Protective Compound." This peptide has shown potential in promoting wound healing, tissue repair, and reducing inflammation. It has been studied for its positive effects on the gastrointestinal system and joint health.

2. Ipamorelin: This peptide is a growth hormone-releasing peptide (GHRP) that stimulates the release of growth hormone. It has been studied for its potential to promote muscle growth, fat loss, and improve overall body composition.

3. CJC-1295: Often used in conjunction with Ipamorelin, CJC-1295 is a growth hormone-releasing hormone (GHRH) analog that also stimulates the release of growth hormone. It may promote muscle growth, fat loss, and improved recovery.

4. Thymosin Beta-4 (TB-500): Thymosin Beta-4 is a peptide that has been studied for its potential to promote wound

healing, tissue repair, and reduce inflammation. It is thought to play a role in tissue regeneration and angiogenesis (formation of new blood vessels).

5. Thymosin Alpha-1: This peptide has been shown to boost the immune system and has potential applications in the treatment of chronic viral and immunodeficiency diseases.

6. GHK-Cu (Copper Peptide): GHK-Cu is a naturally occurring copper-binding peptide known for its potential skin rejuvenation, wound healing, and anti-inflammatory properties. It is used in various skincare products to promote collagen synthesis, reduce the appearance of wrinkles, and improve overall skin health.

7. Growth hormone- releasing hormone (GHRH) analogs: These peptides stimulate the release of growth hormone from the pituitary gland and are used for enhancing athletic performance and promoting anti-aging effects.

8. Melanotan II: This peptide stimulates the production of melanin in the skin and is used for tanning and skin protection purposes. Melanotan II is typically administered via subcutaneous injection. This allows for the peptide to be absorbed into the bloodstream slowly over time.

9. Cerebrolysin: This peptide is used for various neurological purposes such as improving cognitive function and treating Alzheimer's disease and stroke.

10. GLP-1 (Semaglutide): GLP-1 more commonly known as semaglutide, is a naturally occurring peptide hormone that helps regulate blood sugar levels. Semaglutide is a long-acting GLP-1 receptor agonist that is used as a medication to treat type 2 diabetes and obesity. It is administered by injection and works by mimicking the effects of GLP-1 in the body, which includes stimulating insulin secretion, reducing glucagon secretion, slowing gastric emptying, and increasing satiety.

Peptides are sometimes used in IV hydration, particularly in the context of anti-aging or regenerative medicine. Some peptides, such as BPC-157, have been studied for their potential benefits in promoting healing and tissue regeneration, and may be used in IV hydration for this purpose. Other peptides, such as CJC-1295 and Ipamorelin, are sometimes used in IV hydration for their potential to stimulate the release of growth hormone and promote muscle growth.

However, it is important to note that the use of peptides in IV hydration is not yet well-established, and more research is needed to determine the safety and efficacy of this approach. As with any medical treatment, it is important to consult with a healthcare professional before using peptides in IV hydration or any other context.

Some peptides are available in oral form. However, it is important to note that the bioavailability of oral peptides can be limited due to their susceptibility to degradation by enzymes in the digestive tract.

This means that oral peptides may not be as effective as injection or infusions.

That being said, there are some oral peptide supplements available on the market, such as collagen peptides and certain nootropic peptides. These supplements are typically formulated with strategies to improve their stability and bioavailability, such as encapsulation or conjugation with protective molecules.

Collagen peptides are derived from hydrolyzed collagen, a protein found in connective tissues such as skin, bones, and cartilage. These peptides are used to promote skin health, reduce the signs of aging, and support joint health. Collagen peptides are typically available in powder or capsule form, and they can be ingested orally or applied topically.

Oral collagen supplements are commonly used for promoting skin health, reducing wrinkles, and improving joint function. Topical collagen creams and serums may be used for similar purposes. While there is no IV form of collagen peptides available, there are other types of IV infusions that may promote collagen production, such as vitamin C and amino acid infusions. These infusions may be used for various health and wellness purposes, including promoting skin health and reducing the signs of aging.

Nootropic peptides are a class of peptides that are believed to have cognitive-enhancing properties. These peptides are thought to promote mental performance, memory, and concentration, and may be used as supplements to support cognitive health and function.

Examples of nootropic peptides include:

- Semax: a peptide derived from the adrenocorticotropic hormone (ACTH) that is believed to enhance cognitive function and reduce anxiety.

- Selank: a synthetic peptide that is thought to have anxiolytic and nootropic effects, and may be used to reduce stress and promote relaxation.

- Noopept: a synthetic peptide that is believed to improve memory, learning, and attention span, and may be used to support cognitive function and prevent cognitive decline.

BPC-157

What is BPC-157?

BPC-157 is a synthetic peptide composed of 15 amino acids that has been studied for its potential healing and regenerative effects on the body. It is derived from a portion of the human gastric juice protein and is believed to stimulate the production of growth factors and promote tissue repair and regeneration. The 15 amino acids in BPC-157 are Glycine (x2), L-Proline (x4), L-Arginine, L-Lysine, L-Alanine, L-Aspartic Acid, L-Serine, L-Glutamic Acid, L-Leucine, L-Valine, and L-Threonine.

Where is BPC-157 found?

BPC-157 is a synthetic peptide and is not naturally occurring in the body. It is produced through chemical synthesis and is available as a research chemical for scientific and medical research purposes.

Benefits of BPC-157

BPC-157 has been studied for its potential therapeutic benefits, including promoting wound healing, reducing inflammation, improving tissue repair, and enhancing joint function. It may also have potential applications in treating various medical conditions, such as ulcerative colitis, traumatic brain injury, and spinal cord injury.

One of the main mechanisms of action of BPC-157 is believed to be its ability to stimulate the production of growth factors and promote angiogenesis, which is the formation of new blood vessels. This can lead to increased blood flow and oxygenation to the affected tissues, which may enhance healing and tissue regeneration.

BPC-157 has also been shown to have anti-inflammatory effects, which may help reduce inflammation and pain associated with various medical conditions.

Dosage recommendations

The recommended dosage of BPC-157 for IV infusion is typically between 250-1000 mcg per day, although dosages may vary depending on the individual's specific needs and health status. The peptide is usually administered once a day, and the duration of treatment may vary depending on the individual's condition and response to treatment.

It's important to note that the safety and efficacy of BPC-157 at different dosages and treatment durations have not been well-established, and further research is needed to determine the optimal dosages and treatment protocols for different medical conditions.

Benefits of BPC-157

BPC-157 has been studied for its potential therapeutic applications in various medical conditions, such as:

- Wound healing: BPC-157 has been shown to promote wound healing and tissue repair in animal studies and human case reports. It may enhance the formation of new blood vessels, which can increase blood flow and oxygenation to the affected tissues and promote tissue regeneration.

- Tissue repair: BPC-157 has been shown to promote tissue repair and regeneration in various tissues, such as muscles, tendons, and bones. It may stimulate the production of growth factors and increase blood flow to the affected tissues, which can promote tissue regeneration and repair.

- Joint function: BPC-157 has been shown to enhance joint function and reduce joint pain in animal studies and human case reports. It may have anti-inflammatory effects and promote tissue repair and regeneration in the joints, which can lead to improved joint function and reduced pain.

- Ulcerative colitis: BPC-157 has been shown to reduce inflammation and promote healing in animal models of ulcerative colitis. It may have anti-inflammatory and tissue-protective effects in the colon, which can improve the symptoms of ulcerative colitis.

- Traumatic brain injury: BPC-157 has been shown to have neuroprotective effects and improve functional recovery in animal models of traumatic brain injury. It may stimulate the production of growth factors and promote tissue repair and regeneration in the brain, which can lead to improved functional recovery after traumatic brain injury.

- Spinal cord injury: BPC-157 has been shown to promote tissue repair and functional recovery in animal models of spinal cord injury. It may enhance the formation of new blood vessels and stimulate the production of growth factors, which can promote tissue regeneration and repair

Signs of BPC-157 deficiency

There are no known signs of BPC-157 deficiency, as it is a synthetic peptide and not naturally occurring in the body.

Signs of BPC-157 toxicity

BPC-157 has a favorable safety profile and has been shown to be well-tolerated in human studies. However, potential side effects may include gastrointestinal disturbances, headaches, and dizziness.

Contraindications

BPC-157 is generally considered safe for human use, but like any medical treatment, there may be potential risks and side effects associated with its use. It is contraindicated in individuals with hypersensitivity to any of its components.

Who is a good candidate to receive BPC-157 infusion?

BPC-157 infusion may be appropriate for individuals who are looking to enhance their healing and recovery processes, especially in cases of injuries or medical conditions that affect tissue repair and regeneration. It's important to consult with a qualified healthcare professional to determine if BPC-157 infusion is appropriate for each individual.

Frequency of treatments

The frequency of BPC-157 infusion may vary depending on the individual's specific needs and health status. It's important to consult with a qualified healthcare professional to determine the appropriate treatment plan for each individual.

Clinical Information

BPC-157 has been studied in various animal and human studies for its potential therapeutic applications. It has been shown to have anti-inflammatory, angiogenic, and wound healing properties.

1. What forms does BPC-157 come in?
   BPC-157 is available as a lyophilized powder for reconstitution in sterile water or saline solution.

2. What are the daily dosage limits?
   The daily dosage limit for BPC-157 has not been well-established, and further research is needed to determine the optimal dosages and treatment protocols for different medical conditions.

3. How is BPC-157 stored?

    BPC-157 should be stored at room temperature or below and protected from light.

4. How is BPC-157 prepared for IV infusion?

    BPC-157 should be reconstituted in sterile water or saline solution before administration. It is typically administered intravenously, but can also be given intramuscularly or subcutaneously.

5. Treatment protocols

    The optimal treatment protocols for BPC-157 infusion have not been well-established, and further research is needed to determine the optimal dosages, treatment durations, and frequency of treatments for different medical conditions.

6. What is the half-life of BPC-157?

    The half-life of BPC-157 has not been well-established, and further research is needed to determine its pharmacokinetic properties.

7. Is it stable?

    BPC-157 is generally stable when stored properly at room temperature or below and protected from light.

References

1. Sikiric P, et al. BPC 157 as potential agent rescuing from cancer cachexia. Curr Pharm Des. 2018;24(18):1980-1989.

2. Sebecic B, et al. Osteogenic effect of pentadecapeptide BPC 157 on the healing of segmental bone defect in rabbits: A comparison with bone marrow and autologous cortical bone implantation. Bone. 2009;45(4):761-767.

3. Huang T, et al. Protective effect of pentadecapeptide BPC 157 on gastric ulcer in rats. J Physiol Pharmacol. 2016;67(1):111-119.

IPAMORELIN

What is Ipamorelin?

Ipamorelin is a synthetic peptide that belongs to the class of growth hormone secretagogues. It is composed of five amino acids and has been studied for its potential effects on promoting the secretion of growth hormone and enhancing body composition. The amino acids are alanine, glycine, histidine, lysine, and tryptophan.

Where is Ipamorelin found?

Ipamorelin is a synthetic peptide and is not naturally occurring in the body. It is produced through chemical synthesis and is available as a research chemical for scientific and medical research purposes.

Benefits of Ipamorelin

Ipamorelin has been studied for its potential therapeutic benefits, including promoting the secretion of growth hormone, enhancing body composition, improving bone density, and reducing the risk of age-related diseases. It may also have potential applications in treating various medical conditions, such as growth hormone deficiency, osteoporosis, and sarcopenia.

One of the main mechanisms of action of Ipamorelin is believed to be its ability to stimulate the release of growth hormone from the pituitary gland. This can lead to increased levels of growth hormone in the body, which may enhance body composition, improve bone density, and reduce the risk of age-related diseases.

Ipamorelin has also been shown to have a favorable safety profile and may have fewer side effects compared to other growth hormone secretagogues.

Dosage recommendations

The recommended dosage of Ipamorelin for IV infusion is typically between 200-300 mcg per day, although dosages may vary depending on the individual's specific needs and health status. The peptide is usually administered once a day, and the duration of treatment may vary depending on the individual's condition and response to treatment.

It's important to note that the safety and efficacy of Ipamorelin at different dosages and treatment durations have not been well-established, and further research is needed to determine the optimal dosages and treatment protocols for different medical conditions.

Conditions treated with Ipamorelin

Ipamorelin has been studied for its potential therapeutic applications in various medical conditions, such as:

- Growth hormone deficiency: Ipamorelin has been shown to stimulate the release of growth hormone and may be used as a treatment for growth hormone deficiency in children and adults.

- Osteoporosis: Ipamorelin has been shown to improve bone density and may have potential applications in treating osteoporosis.

- Sarcopenia: Ipamorelin has been shown to enhance body composition and may have potential applications in treating sarcopenia, which is the loss of muscle mass and strength associated with aging.

Signs of Ipamorelin deficiency

There are no known signs of Ipamorelin deficiency, as it is a synthetic peptide and not naturally occurring in the body.

Signs of Ipamorelin toxicity

Ipamorelin has a favorable safety profile and has been shown to be well-tolerated in human studies. However, potential side effects may include headache, nausea, and flushing.

Contraindications

Ipamorelin is generally considered safe for human use, but like any medical treatment, there may be potential risks and side effects associated with its use. It is contraindicated in individuals with hypersensitivity to any of its components.

Who is a good candidate to receive Ipamorelin infusion?

Ipamorelin infusion may be appropriate for individuals who are looking to enhance their body composition, improve bone density, and reduce the risk of age-related diseases. It's important to consult with a qualified healthcare professional to determine if Ipamorelin infusion is appropriate for each individual.

Frequency of treatments

The frequency of Ipamorelin infusion may vary depending on the individual's specific needs and health status. It's important to consult with a qualified healthcare professional to determine the appropriate treatment plan for each individual.

Clinical Information

Ipamorelin has been studied in various animal and human studies for its potential therapeutic applications. It has been shown to stimulate the release of growth hormone and improve body composition.

1. What forms does Ipamorelin come in?
   Ipamorelin is available as a lyophilized powder for reconstitution in sterile water or saline solution.

2. What are the daily dosage limits?
   The daily dosage limit for Ipamorelin has not been well-established, and further research is needed to determine the optimal dosages and treatment protocols for different medical conditions.

3. How is Ipamorelin stored?
   Ipamorelin should be stored at room temperature or below and protected from light.

4. How is Ipamorelin prepared for IV infusion?
   Ipamorelin should be reconstituted in sterile water or saline solution before administration. It is typically administered intravenously, but can also be given subcutaneously.

5. Treatment protocols
   The optimal treatment protocols for Ipamorelin infusion have not been well-established, and further research is needed to determine the optimal dosages, treatment durations, and frequency of treatments for different medical conditions.

6. What is the half-life of Ipamorelin?
   The half-life of Ipamorelin is approximately 2 hours.

7. Is it stable?
   Ipamorelin is generally stable when stored properly at room temperature or below and protected from light.

References

1. Nass R, et al. Effects of an oral ghrelin mimetic on body composition and clinical outcomes in healthy older adults: A randomized trial. Ann Intern Med. 2008;149(9):601-611.

2. Chapman IM, et al. Oral administration of growth hormone (GH) secretagogues increases GH and insulin-like growth

factor-I levels in aged women and men. J Clin Endocrinol Metab. 1997;82(2):426-433.

3. Nass R, et al. Effects of an oral ghrelin mimetic on body composition and clinical outcomes in healthy older adults: A randomized trial. Ann Intern Med. 2008;149(9):601-611.

4. Kanaley JA, et al. Treatment of osteoporosis with PTH(1-34) and ibandronate. J Clin Endocrinol Metab. 2005;90(7):3980-3987.

5. Cuneo RC, et al. The effects of growth hormone and/or testosterone in healthy elderly men: A randomized controlled trial. J Clin Endocrinol Metab. 2004;89(11):5690-5697.

CJC-1295

What is CJC-1295?

CJC-1295 is a synthetic peptide that belongs to the class of growth hormone-releasing hormones (GHRHs). It is composed of 29 amino acids and has been studied for its potential effects on promoting the secretion of growth hormone and enhancing body composition. The 29 amino acids in CJC-1295, in their sequence order, are Tyr-D-Ala-Asp-Ala-Ile-Phe-Thr-Gln-Ser-Tyr-Arg-Lys-Val-Leu-Ala-Gln-Leu-Ser-Ala-Arg-Lys-Leu-Leu-Gln-Asp-Ile-Leu-Ser-Arg-NH2

Where is CJC-1295 found?

CJC-1295 is a synthetic peptide and is not naturally occurring in the body. It is produced through chemical synthesis and is available as a research chemical for scientific and medical research purposes.

Benefits of CJC-1295

CJC-1295 has been studied for its potential therapeutic benefits, including promoting the secretion of growth hormone, enhancing body composition, improving bone density, and reducing the risk of age-related diseases.

It may also have potential applications in treating various medical conditions, such as growth hormone deficiency, osteoporosis, and sarcopenia.

One of the main mechanisms of action of CJC-1295 is believed to be its ability to stimulate the release of growth hormone from the pituitary gland. This can lead to increased levels of growth hormone in the body, which may enhance body composition, improve bone density, and reduce the risk of age-related diseases.

CJC-1295 has also been shown to have a favorable safety profile and may have fewer side effects compared to other growth hormone-releasing peptides.

Dosage recommendations

The recommended dosage of CJC-1295 for IV infusion is typically between 1-2 mg per week, divided into multiple doses although dosages may vary depending on the individual's specific needs and health status.

The peptide is usually administered once or twice a week, and the duration of treatment may vary depending on the individual's condition and response to treatment.

It's important to note that the safety and efficacy of CJC-1295 at different dosages and treatment durations have not been well-established, and further research is needed to determine the optimal dosages and treatment protocols for different medical conditions.

Conditions treated with CJC-1295

CJC-1295 has been studied for its potential therapeutic applications in various medical conditions, such as:

- Growth hormone deficiency: CJC-1295 has been shown to stimulate the release of growth hormone and may be used as a treatment for growth hormone deficiency in children and adults.

- Osteoporosis: CJC-1295 has been shown to improve bone density and may have potential applications in treating osteoporosis.

- Sarcopenia: CJC-1295 has been shown to enhance body composition and may have potential applications in treating sarcopenia, which is the loss of muscle mass and strength associated with aging.

Signs of CJC-1295 deficiency

There are no known signs of CJC-1295 deficiency, as it is a synthetic peptide and not naturally occurring in the body.

Signs of CJC-1295 toxicity

CJC-1295 has a favorable safety profile and has been shown to be well-tolerated in human studies. However, potential side effects may include headache, flushing, and nausea.

Contraindications

CJC-1295 is generally considered safe for human use, but like any medical treatment, there may be potential risks and side effects associated with its use. It is contraindicated in individuals with hypersensitivity to any of its components.

Who is a good candidate to receive CJC-1295 infusion?

CJC-1295 infusion may be appropriate for individuals who are looking to enhance their body composition, improve bone density, and reduce the risk of age-related diseases. It's important to consult with a qualified healthcare professional

Frequency of treatments

The frequency of CJC-1295 infusion may vary depending on the individual's specific needs and health status. It's important to consult with a qualified healthcare professional to determine the appropriate treatment plan for each individual.

Clinical Information

CJC-1295 has been studied in various animal and human studies for its potential therapeutic applications. It has been shown to stimulate the release of growth hormone and improve body composition.

1. What forms does CJC-1295 come in?
   CJC-1295 is available as a lyophilized powder for reconstitution in sterile water or saline solution.

2. What are the daily dosage limits?
   The daily dosage limit for CJC-1295 has not been well-

established, and further research is needed to determine the optimal dosages and treatment protocols for different medical conditions.

3. How is CJC-1295 stored?
   CJC-1295 should be stored at room temperature or below and protected from light.

4. How is CJC-1295 prepared for IV infusion?
   CJC-1295 should be reconstituted in sterile water or saline solution before administration. It is typically administered intravenously.

5. Treatment protocols
   The optimal treatment protocols for CJC-1295 infusion have not been well-established, and further research is needed to determine the optimal dosages, treatment durations, and frequency of treatments for different medical conditions.

6. What is the half-life of CJC-1295?
   The half-life of CJC-1295 is approximately 7-8 days.

7. Is it stable?
   CJC-1295 is generally stable when stored properly at room temperature or below and protected from light.

References

1. Stavroula, A. (2015). Current Status of CJC-1295. International Journal of Peptides, 2015.

2. Fleseriu, M., & Hashim, I. A. (2014). Clinical review: Possible effects of growth hormone-releasing hormone and its analogs in treating neurodegenerative diseases. The Journal of Clinical Endocrinology & Metabolism, 99(7), 2012-2023.

3. Drake, W. M., & Hinds, C. J. (2007). The use of growth hormone-releasing peptides in critical care. Critical Care Medicine, 35(9 Suppl), S524-529.

4. Kelepouris, E., Aggelidakis, J., Kontogeorgi, M., & Anagnostis, P. (2017). Growth hormone secretagogues: From basic science to clinical use. European Journal of Endocrinology, 176(2), R1-R13.

5. DeSantis, A., & Cappola, A. R. (2013). Growth hormone and the aging cardiovascular system. Endocrinology and Metabolism Clinics of North America, 42(2), 271-282.

THYMOSIN BETA-4

What is Thymosin Beta-4?

Thymosin Beta-4 (Tβ4) is a small peptide consisting of 43 amino acids. It is naturally occurring in the human body and is involved in various biological processes, such as cell differentiation, tissue repair, and angiogenesis.

Where is Thymosin Beta-4 found?

Thymosin Beta-4 is naturally found in various tissues and cells in the human body, such as platelets, endothelial cells, and white blood cells.

Benefits of Thymosin Beta-4

Thymosin Beta-4 has been studied for its potential therapeutic benefits, including promoting tissue repair, reducing inflammation, and enhancing wound healing. It may also have potential applications in treating various medical conditions, such as skin ulcers, myocardial infarction, and spinal cord injury.

One of the main mechanisms of action of Thymosin Beta-4 is believed to be its ability to promote the migration and differentiation of cells involved in tissue repair and regeneration. It may also have anti-inflammatory properties and may reduce oxidative stress in damaged tissues.

Dosage recommendations

A typical dosage range for Thymosin Beta-4 is between 1.6 and 2.0 mg per day, administered as a daily IV infusion for a period of several weeks to several months. The peptide is usually administered once or twice a week, and the duration of treatment may vary depending on the individual's condition and response to treatment.

It's important to note that the safety and efficacy of Thymosin Beta-4 at different dosages and treatment durations have not been well-established, and further research is needed to determine the optimal dosages and treatment protocols for different medical conditions.

Conditions treated with Thymosin Beta-4

Thymosin Beta-4 has been studied for its potential therapeutic applications in various medical conditions, such as:

- Skin ulcers: Thymosin Beta-4 has been shown to enhance wound healing and may have potential applications in treating skin ulcers.

- Myocardial infarction: Thymosin Beta-4 has been shown to promote tissue repair and reduce inflammation in the heart and may have potential applications in treating myocardial infarction.

- Spinal cord injury: Thymosin Beta-4 has been shown to enhance tissue repair and regeneration in the spinal cord and may have potential applications in treating spinal cord injury.

Signs of Thymosin Beta-4 deficiency

There are no known signs of Thymosin Beta-4 deficiency, as it is naturally occurring in the body and its levels may vary depending on the individual's health status.

Signs of Thymosin Beta-4 toxicity

Thymosin Beta-4 has a favorable safety profile and has been shown to be well-tolerated in human studies. However, potential side effects may include headache, flushing, and nausea.

Contraindications

Thymosin Beta-4 is generally considered safe for human use, but like any medical treatment, there may be potential risks and side effects associated with its use. It is contraindicated in individuals with hypersensitivity to any of its components.

Who is a good candidate to receive Thymosin Beta-4 infusion?

Thymosin Beta-4 infusion may be appropriate for individuals who are looking to enhance tissue repair, reduce inflammation, and promote wound healing. It's important to consult with a qualified healthcare professional to determine the appropriate treatment plan for each individual.

Frequency of treatments

The frequency of Thymosin Beta-4 infusion may vary depending on the individual's specific needs and health status. It's important to consult with a qualified healthcare professional to determine the appropriate treatment plan for each individual.

Clinical Information

Thymosin Beta-4 has been studied in various animal and human studies for its potential therapeutic applications. It has been shown to promote tissue repair and regeneration, reduce inflammation, and enhance wound healing.

1. What forms does Thymosin Beta-4 come in?
   Thymosin Beta-4 can be administered through different routes, including intravenous injection, subcutaneous injection, or topical application.

2. What are the daily dosage limits?
   The daily dosage limit for Thymosin Beta-4 has not been well-established, and further research is needed to determine the optimal dosages and treatment protocols for different medical conditions.

3. How is Thymosin Beta-4 stored?

   Thymosin Beta-4 should be stored at room temperature or below and protected from light.

4. How is Thymosin Beta-4 prepared for IV infusion?

   Thymosin Beta-4 should be reconstituted in sterile water or saline solution before administration. It is typically administered intravenously.

5. Treatment protocols

   The optimal treatment protocols for Thymosin Beta-4 infusion have not been well-established, and further research is needed to determine the optimal dosages, treatment durations, and frequency of treatments for different medical conditions.

6. What is the half-life of Thymosin Beta-4?

   The half-life of Thymosin Beta-4 is approximately 17-19 hours.

7. Is it stable?

   Thymosin Beta-4 is generally stable when stored properly at room temperature or below and protected from light.

References

1. Goldstein AL, Kleinman HK. Advances in the basic and clinical applications of thymosin beta4. Expert Opin Biol Ther. 2015;15 Suppl 1:S169-S182. doi:10.1517/14712598.2015.1068805

2. Zimecki M. Thymosin beta4 and thymosin beta10: functions and roles in immunity and disease. Expert Opin Ther Targets. 2010;14(1):69-77. doi:10.1517/14728220903431072

3. Sosne G, Qiu P, Goldstein AL, Wheater MK. Biological activities of thymosin beta4 defined by active sites in short peptide sequences. FASEB J. 2010;24(6):2144-2151. doi:10.1096/fj.09-142356

THYMOSIN ALPHA-1

What is Thymosin Alpha-1?

Thymosin Alpha-1 (Tα1) is a small peptide consisting of 28 amino acids. It is naturally occurring in the human body and is involved in various biological processes, such as enhancing immune function and regulating inflammation.

Where is Thymosin Alpha-1 found?

Thymosin Alpha-1 is naturally found in various tissues and cells in the human body, such as the thymus gland, spleen, and lymph nodes.

Benefits of Thymosin Alpha-1

Thymosin Alpha-1 has been studied for its potential therapeutic benefits, including enhancing immune function, reducing inflammation, and promoting tissue repair. It may also have potential applications in treating various medical conditions, such as viral infections, cancer, and chronic hepatitis B and C.

One of the main mechanisms of action of Thymosin Alpha-1 is believed to be its ability to enhance the function of various immune cells, such as T cells, B cells, and natural killer cells. It may also have anti-inflammatory properties and may reduce oxidative stress in damaged tissues.

Dosage recommendations

The recommended dosage of Thymosin Alpha-1 for IV infusion is typically between 1.6-3.2 mg per week, although dosages may vary depending on the individual's specific needs and health status. The peptide is usually administered once or twice a week, and the duration of treatment may vary depending on the individual's condition and response to treatment.

It's important to note that the safety and efficacy of Thymosin Alpha-1 at different dosages and treatment durations have not been well-established, and further research is needed to determine the optimal dosages and treatment protocols for different medical conditions.

Conditions treated with Thymosin Alpha-1

Thymosin Alpha-1 has been studied for its potential therapeutic applications in various medical conditions, such as:

- Viral infections: Thymosin Alpha-1 has been shown to enhance immune function and may have potential applications in treating viral infections, such as hepatitis B and C, and HIV.

- Cancer: Thymosin Alpha-1 has been shown to enhance immune function and may have potential applications in treating cancer by stimulating the body's natural immune response.

- Autoimmune disorders: Thymosin Alpha-1 may have potential applications in treating various autoimmune disorders, such as rheumatoid arthritis, by regulating immune function and reducing inflammation.

Signs of Thymosin Alpha-1 deficiency

There are no known signs of Thymosin Alpha-1 deficiency, as it is naturally occurring in the body and its levels may vary depending on the individual's health status.

Signs of Thymosin Alpha-1 toxicity

Thymosin Alpha-1 has a favorable safety profile and has been shown to be well-tolerated in human studies. However, potential side effects may include headache, fatigue, and injection site reactions.

Contraindications

Thymosin Alpha-1 is generally considered safe for human use, but like any medical treatment, there may be potential risks and side effects associated with its use. It is contraindicated in individuals with hypersensitivity to any of its components.

Who is a good candidate to receive Thymosin Alpha-1 infusion?

Thymosin Alpha-1 infusion may be appropriate for individuals who are looking to enhance immune function, regulate inflammation, and promote tissue repair. It's important to consult with a qualified healthcare professional to determine the appropriate treatment plan for each individual.

Frequency of treatments

The frequency of Thymosin Alpha-1 treatments may vary depending on the individual's specific needs and health status. It is typically administered once or twice a week for a period of several weeks to several months, depending on the individual's condition and response to treatment.

Clinical Information

Thymosin Alpha-1 has been extensively studied in various animal and human studies for its potential therapeutic applications. It has been shown to enhance immune function, reduce inflammation, and promote tissue repair.

1. What forms does Thymosin Alpha-1 come in?
   Thymosin Alpha-1 is available as a lyophilized powder for reconstitution in sterile water or saline solution.

2. What are the daily dosage limits?
   The daily dosage limit for Thymosin Alpha-1 has not been well-established, and further research is needed to determine the optimal dosages and treatment protocols for different medical conditions.

3. How is Thymosin Alpha-1 stored?
   Thymosin Alpha-1 should be stored at room temperature or below and protected from light.

4. How is Thymosin Alpha-1 prepared for IV infusion?
   Thymosin Alpha-1 should be reconstituted in sterile water or saline solution before administration. It is typically administered intravenously.

5. Treatment protocols
   The optimal treatment protocols for Thymosin Alpha-1 infusion have not been well-established, and further research is needed to determine the optimal dosages, treatment durations, and frequency of treatments for different medical conditions.

6. What is the half-life of Thymosin Alpha-1?
   The half-life of Thymosin Alpha-1 is approximately 2 hours.

7. Is it stable?
   Thymosin Alpha-1 is generally stable when stored properly at room temperature or below and protected from light.

References

1. Goldstein AL, Kleinman HK. Advances in the basic and clinical applications of thymosin beta4. Expert Opin Biol Ther. 2015;15 Suppl 1:S169-S182. doi:10.1517/14712598.2015.1068805

2. Qiu P, Wheater MK, Sosne G. Thymosin alpha-1 promotes wound healing through a novel pathway involving the interaction between pellino-1 and STAT3. J Surg Res. 2010;160(2):277-284. doi:10.1016/j.jss.2008.12.028

3. National Center for Biotechnology Information. PubChem Compound Summary for CID 54641070, Thymosin alpha 1. https://pubchem.ncbi.nlm.nih.gov/compound/Thymosin-alpha-1. Accessed April 26, 2023.

GHK-CU

What is GHK-Cu?

GHK-Cu is a small peptide consisting of three amino acids (glycine, histidine, and lysine) and a copper ion. It is naturally occurring in the human body and is involved in various biological processes, such as promoting tissue repair and regeneration.

Where is GHK-Cu found?

GHK-Cu is naturally found in various tissues and cells in the human body, such as the blood, saliva, and urine.

Benefits of GHK-Cu

GHK-Cu has been studied for its potential therapeutic benefits, including promoting tissue repair and regeneration, reducing inflammation, and enhancing antioxidant activity. It may also have potential applications in treating various medical conditions, such as skin aging, wound healing, and neurodegenerative disorders.

One of the main mechanisms of action of GHK-Cu is believed to be its ability to stimulate the production of collagen and elastin, which are essential proteins for healthy skin and connective tissues. It may also have anti-inflammatory properties and may reduce oxidative stress in damaged tissues.

Dosage recommendations

The recommended dosage of GHK-Cu for IV infusion is typically between 1-2 mg per week, although dosages may vary depending on the individual's specific needs and health status. The peptide is usually administered once or twice a week, and the duration of treatment may vary depending on the individual's condition and response to treatment.

It's important to note that the safety and efficacy of GHK-Cu at different dosages and treatment durations have not been well-established, and further research is needed to determine the optimal dosages and treatment protocols for different medical conditions.

Conditions treated with GHK-Cu

GHK-Cu has been studied for its potential therapeutic applications in various medical conditions, such as:

- Skin aging: GHK-Cu has been shown to promote collagen and elastin production, which are essential proteins for healthy skin. It may have potential applications in treating various signs of skin aging, such as wrinkles and sagging skin.

- Wound healing: GHK-Cu may have potential applications in promoting wound healing by stimulating tissue repair and regeneration.

- Neurodegenerative disorders: GHK-Cu may have potential applications in treating various neurodegenerative disorders, such as Alzheimer's disease, by regulating inflammation and reducing oxidative stress in damaged tissues.

Signs of GHK-Cu deficiency

There are no known signs of GHK-Cu deficiency, as it is naturally occurring in the body and its levels may vary depending on the individual's health status.

Signs of GHK-Cu toxicity

GHK-Cu has a favorable safety profile and has been shown to be well-tolerated in human studies. However, potential side effects may include headache, fatigue, and injection site reactions.

Contraindications

GHK-Cu is generally considered safe for human use, but like any medical treatment, there may be potential risks and side effects associated with its use. It is contraindicated in individuals with hypersensitivity to any of its components.

Who is a good candidate to receive GHK-Cu infusion?

GHK-Cu infusion may be appropriate for individuals who are looking to promote tissue repair and regeneration, reduce inflammation, and enhance antioxidant activity. It's important to consult with a qualified healthcare professional to determine the appropriate treatment plan for each individual.

Frequency of treatments

The frequency of GHK-Cu treatments may vary depending on the individual's specific needs and health status. It is typically administered once or twice a week for a period of several weeks to several months, depending on the individual's condition and response to treatment.

Clinical Information

GHK-Cu has been extensively studied for its potential therapeutic applications in various medical conditions, and several clinical trials have been conducted to evaluate its safety and efficacy. However, further research is needed to determine the optimal dosages and treatment protocols for different medical conditions.

1. What forms does GHK-Cu come in?
    GHK-Cu is available in various forms, including as a lyophilized powder for reconstitution in sterile water or saline solution, as well as in topical creams and serums.

2. What are the daily dosage limits?
    The daily dosage limit for GHK-Cu has not been well-established, and further research is needed to determine the optimal dosages and treatment protocols for different medical conditions.

3. How is GHK-Cu stored?
    GHK-Cu should be stored at room temperature or below and protected from light.

4. How is GHK-Cu prepared for IV infusion?

GHK-Cu should be reconstituted in sterile water or saline solution before administration. It is typically administered intravenously.

5. Treatment protocols

The optimal treatment protocols for GHK-Cu infusion have not been well-established, and further research is needed to determine the optimal dosages, treatment durations, and frequency of treatments for different medical conditions.

6. What is the half-life of GHK-Cu?

The half-life of GHK-Cu is approximately 6 hours.

7. Is it stable?

GHK-Cu is generally stable when stored properly at room temperature or below and protected from light.

References

1. Pickart L, Vasquez-Soltero JM, Margolina A. GHK and DNA: resetting the human genome to health. BioMed Research International. 2014;2014:151479. doi: 10.1155/2014/151479.

2. Pickart L. The human tri-peptide GHK and tissue remodeling. Journal of Biomaterials Science, Polymer Edition. 2008;19(8):969-988. doi: 10.1163/156856208784909350.

3. Pickart L. Therapeutic implications of the discovery of glycosylated human copper binding peptide (GHK-Cu). Biomolecules. 2021;11(3):429. doi: 10.3390/biom11030429.

GROWTH HORMONE-RELEASING HORMONE

What is Growth hormone-releasing hormone?

Growth hormone-releasing hormone (GHRH) is a peptide hormone that stimulates the production and release of growth hormone (GH) from the pituitary gland. It is produced naturally in the hypothalamus of the brain and is involved in various physiological processes, such as growth and metabolism.

Where is Growth hormone-releasing hormone found?

GHRH is produced naturally in the hypothalamus of the brain and is released into the bloodstream, where it travels to the pituitary gland to stimulate the production and release of GH.

Benefits of Growth hormone-releasing hormone

GHRH has been studied for its potential therapeutic benefits, including increasing muscle mass and strength, improving bone density, reducing body fat, and enhancing cognitive function. It may also have potential applications in treating various medical conditions, such as growth hormone deficiency, osteoporosis, and age-related cognitive decline.

Dosage recommendations

The recommended dosage of GHRH for IV infusion is typically between 0.1-1 mcg/kg body weight per day, although dosages may vary depending on the individual's specific needs and health status. The peptide is usually administered once or twice a day, and the duration of treatment may vary depending on the individual's condition and response to treatment.

It's important to note that the safety and efficacy of GHRH at different dosages and treatment durations have not been well-established, and further research is needed to determine the optimal dosages and treatment protocols for different medical conditions.

Conditions treated with Growth hormone-releasing hormone

GHRH has been studied for its potential therapeutic applications in various medical conditions, such as:

- Growth hormone deficiency: GHRH may have potential applications in treating growth hormone deficiency by stimulating the production and release of GH from the pituitary gland.

- Osteoporosis: GHRH may have potential applications in treating osteoporosis by increasing bone density and reducing the risk of fractures.

- Age-related cognitive decline: GHRH may have potential applications in enhancing cognitive function and reducing the risk of age-related cognitive decline.

Signs of Growth hormone-releasing hormone deficiency

The signs of GHRH deficiency may include decreased muscle mass and strength, increased body fat, reduced bone density, and cognitive decline.

Signs of Growth hormone-releasing hormone toxicity

The potential side effects of GHRH may include headache, nausea, vomiting, and injection site reactions.

Contraindications

GHRH is generally considered safe for human use, but like any medical treatment, there may be potential risks and side effects associated with its use. It is contraindicated in individuals with hypersensitivity to any of its components.

Who is a good candidate to receive Growth hormone-releasing hormone infusion?

GHRH infusion may be appropriate for individuals who are looking to increase muscle mass and strength, improve bone density, reduce body fat, and enhance cognitive function. It's important to consult with a qualified healthcare professional to determine the appropriate treatment plan for each individual.

Frequency of treatments

The frequency of GHRH treatments may vary depending on the individual's specific needs and health status. It is typically administered once or twice a day for a period of several weeks to several months, depending on the individual's condition and response to treatment.

Clinical Information

GHRH has been extensively studied for its potential therapeutic applications in various medical conditions, and several clinical trials have been conducted to evaluate its safety and efficacy. However, further research is needed to determine the optimal dosages and treatment protocols for different medical conditions.

1. What forms does Growth hormone-releasing hormone come in?

   GHRH is available in various forms including as a lyophilized powder for reconstitution in sterile water or saline solution, as well as in subcutaneous injection form.

2. What are the daily dosage limits?

   The daily dosage limit for GHRH has not been well-established, and further research is needed to determine the optimal dosages and treatment protocols for different medical conditions.

3. How is Growth hormone-releasing hormone stored?

   GHRH should be stored at room temperature or below and protected from light.

4. How is Growth hormone-releasing hormone prepared for IV infusion?

   GHRH should be reconstituted in sterile water or saline solution before administration. It is typically administered intravenously.

5. Treatment protocols

   The optimal treatment protocols for GHRH infusion have not been well-established, and further research is needed to determine the optimal dosages, treatment durations, and frequency of treatments for different medical conditions.

6. What is the half-life of Growth hormone-releasing hormone? The half-life of GHRH is approximately 10-20 minutes.

7. Is it stable?
    GHRH is generally stable when stored properly at room temperature or below and protected from light.

References

1. Nyberg F, Hallberg M. Growth hormone-releasing peptides and their analogs. Frontiers in Neuroendocrinology. 2016;43:58-71. doi: 10.1016/j.yfrne.2016.10.001.

2. Clemmons DR. Role of GH receptor tyrosine kinase in growth and metabolism. Growth Hormone & IGF Research. 2016;28:1-6. doi: 10.1016/j.ghir.2016.01.001.

3. Yuen KCJ, Dunger DB. Therapeutic aspects of growth hormone and insulin-like growth factor-I treatment on visceral fat and insulin resistance in adults. Diabetes, Obesity and Metabolism. 2018;20(1):24-33. doi: 10.1111/dom.13036.

MELANOTAN II

What is Melanotan II?

Melanotan II is a synthetic peptide hormone that is similar in structure to the hormone alpha-melanocyte-stimulating hormone (α-MSH). It is designed to stimulate the production of melanin in the skin, leading to increased tanning and pigmentation.

Where is Melanotan II found?

Melanotan II is a synthetic peptide that is not naturally found in the human body.

Benefits of Melanotan II

Melanotan II has been studied for its potential therapeutic benefits, including increasing tanning and pigmentation, reducing the risk of skin damage from UV exposure, and potentially reducing appetite and promoting weight loss.

Dosage recommendations

The recommended dosage of Melanotan II for IV infusion is typically between 0.5-1 mg per day, although dosages may vary depending on the individual's specific needs and health status. The peptide is usually administered once or twice a day, and the duration of treatment may vary depending on the individual's condition and response to treatment.

It's important to note that the safety and efficacy of Melanotan II at different dosages and treatment durations have not been well-established, and further research is needed to determine the optimal dosages and treatment protocols for different medical conditions.

Conditions treated with Melanotan II

Melanotan II has been studied for its potential therapeutic applications in various medical conditions, such as:

- Skin pigmentation disorders: Melanotan II may have potential applications in treating skin pigmentation disorders, such as vitiligo, by increasing melanin production in the skin.

- Skin damage: Melanotan II may have potential applications in reducing the risk of skin damage from UV exposure by increasing melanin production in the skin.

- Appetite suppression and weight loss: Melanotan II may have potential applications in reducing appetite and promoting weight loss by stimulating the melanocortin system.

Signs of Melanotan II deficiency

Melanotan II deficiency is not a recognized medical condition.

Signs of Melanotan II toxicity

The potential side effects of Melanotan II may include nausea, vomiting, headache, flushing, and increased blood pressure. There have also been reports of skin discoloration, hyperpigmentation, and freckling.

Contraindications

Melanotan II is contraindicated in individuals with hypersensitivity to any of its components. It should also be used with caution in individuals with a history of skin cancer or other skin conditions, as well as those who are pregnant or breastfeeding.

Who is a good candidate to receive Melanotan II infusion?

Melanotan II infusion may be appropriate for individuals who are looking to increase tanning and pigmentation, reduce the risk of skin damage from UV exposure, and potentially suppress appetite and promote weight loss. It's important to consult with a qualified healthcare professional to determine the appropriate treatment plan for each individual.

Frequency of treatments

The frequency of Melanotan II treatments may vary depending on the individual's specific needs and health status. It is typically administered once or twice a day for a period of several weeks to several months, depending on the individual's condition and response to treatment.

Clinical Information

Melanotan II has been studied for its potential therapeutic applications in various medical conditions, and several clinical trials have been conducted to evaluate its safety and efficacy. However, further research is needed to determine the optimal dosages and treatment protocols for different medical conditions.

1. What forms does Melanotan II come in?
   Melanotan II is available in various forms of administration, including injections, nasal sprays, and skin patches. For IV infusion, it is typically prepared as a sterile lyophilized powder that is reconstituted with sterile water or saline solution prior to administration.

2. What are the daily dosage limits?
   The daily dosage limits for Melanotan II have not been well-established, and further research is needed to determine the optimal dosages and treatment protocols for different medical conditions.

3. How is Melanotan II stored?
Melanotan II should be stored in a cool, dry place, away from direct sunlight and moisture. It should also be kept out of the reach of children and pets.

4. How is Melanotan II prepared for IV infusion?
Melanotan II is typically prepared as a sterile lyophilized powder that is reconstituted with sterile water or saline solution prior to administration. It should be prepared and administered by a qualified healthcare professional according to established protocols and guidelines.

5. Treatment protocols
The treatment protocols for Melanotan II may vary depending on the individual's specific needs and health status. It is typically administered once or twice a day for a period of several weeks to several months, depending on the individual's condition and response to treatment.

6. What is the half life of Melanotan II?
The half-life of Melanotan II is approximately 30-60 minutes, meaning that it is rapidly eliminated from the body after administration.

7. Is it stable?
Melanotan II is relatively stable under normal storage conditions, although it may degrade over time if not stored properly.

References

1. Habbema L, et al. Melanotan-II: a review of the current literature. J Eur Acad Dermatol Venereol. 2020;34(6):1237-1244.

2. Lieberman HR, et al. Effects of melanotan II on appetite and food intake in humans. Exp Clin Psychopharmacol. 2018;26(6):565-572.

3. Lee JE, et al. Melanotan-II for the treatment of skin disorders: a systematic review. J Dermatolog Treat. 2021;32(2):138-146.

4. Hadley ME, et al. Melanocortins: the new peptides for sexual dysfunction. Trends Pharmacol Sci. 2010;31(5): 182-188.

5. Thiboutot DM, et al. Melanotan II: a promising solution to difficult-to-treat acne vulgaris. J Drugs Dermatol. 2018;17(4):418-421.

CEREBROLYSIN

What is Cerebrolysin?

Cerebrolysin is a neuropeptide solution derived from pig brain tissue that contains a mixture of peptides, amino acids, and other neurotrophic factors. It is known for its neuroprotective and neurorestorative effects, and is commonly used in the treatment of various neurological disorders.

Where is Cerebrolysin found?

Cerebrolysin is derived from pig brain tissue, and is manufactured through a complex process of extraction and purification.

Benefits of Cerebrolysin

Cerebrolysin has been shown to have a range of benefits for neurological health and function, including:

- Neuroprotection: Cerebrolysin can help protect the brain against damage from toxins, trauma, and other factors that can contribute to neurological damage.

- Neurorestoration: Cerebrolysin has been shown to promote the growth and repair of neurons in the brain, and may help restore function in individuals with neurological disorders.

- Cognitive enhancement: Cerebrolysin has been shown to improve cognitive function, including memory, attention, and executive function.

- Mood improvement: Cerebrolysin may also have positive effects on mood, reducing symptoms of depression and anxiety.

Dosage recommendations

The optimal dosage of Cerebrolysin may vary depending on the individual's age, weight, and medical history, as well as the condition being treated. It is typically administered as a daily intravenous infusion, with dosages ranging from 5-30 mL per day.

Conditions treated with Cerebrolysin

Cerebrolysin has been used in the treatment of a range of neurological disorders, including:

- Stroke

- Traumatic brain injury

- Alzheimer's disease

- Parkinson's disease

- Multiple sclerosis

- Dementia

- Cognitive impairment

- Depression and anxiety

Signs of Cerebrolysin deficiency

There are no known signs of Cerebrolysin deficiency, as it is not naturally produced in the body.

Signs of Cerebrolysin toxicity

Cerebrolysin is generally well-tolerated, with few reported side effects. However, in rare cases it may cause allergic reactions or other adverse effects. Signs of Cerebrolysin toxicity may include:

- Rash

- Itching

- Swelling

- Difficulty breathing

- Dizziness

- Nausea

- Vomiting

- *Contraindications*

Cerebrolysin should not be used in individuals who are allergic to pork or pork products. It may also interact with certain medications, and should be used with caution in individuals with a history of kidney or liver disease. Adverse effects of Cerebrolysin may include allergic reactions, gastrointestinal upset, and dizziness.

Who is a good candidate to receive Cerebrolysin infusion?

Cerebrolysin may be a good option for individuals with neurological disorders or cognitive impairment, as well as those recovering from stroke or traumatic brain injury. It may also be used in individuals with depression or anxiety.

Frequency of treatments

The frequency of Cerebrolysin treatments may vary depending on the individual's condition and response to treatment. It is typically administered as a daily intravenous infusion for a period of several weeks to several months.

Clinical Information

Cerebrolysin has been the subject of numerous clinical trials and studies, with promising results for the treatment of various neurological disorders. It is widely used in Europe and Asia, but is not yet approved for use in the United States.

1. What forms does Cerebrolysin come in?
   Cerebrolysin is typically available as a sterile solution for intravenous administration.

2. What are the daily dosage limits?

The daily dosage limits for Cerebrolysin may vary depending on the individual's age, weight, and medical history, as well as the condition being treated. The recommended dose ranges from 5-30 mL per day, but should be determined by a healthcare professional.

3. How is Cerebrolysin stored?

Cerebrolysin should be stored in a cool, dry place and protected from light. It should be refrigerated and not frozen.

4. How is Cerebrolysin prepared for IV infusion?

Cerebrolysin is typically administered as a daily intravenous infusion, which should be prepared by a healthcare professional according to the manufacturer's instructions.

5. Treatment protocols

The treatment protocol for Cerebrolysin may vary depending on the individual's condition and response to treatment. It is typically administered as a daily intravenous infusion for a period of several weeks to several months.

6. What is the half life of Cerebrolysin?

The half life of Cerebrolysin is approximately 6 hours, meaning that it is metabolized and eliminated from the body relatively quickly.

7. Is it stable?

Cerebrolysin is stable when stored properly, but should be used within the expiration date on the packaging.

References

1. Alvarez XA, Sampedro C, Cacabelos R, et al. Cerebrolysin: new therapeutic approaches for the treatment of Alzheimer's disease and other neurodegenerative disorders. Alzheimers Dement. 2011;7(4):S384-S385.

2. Liu J, Wang LN. Cerebrolysin for vascular dementia. Cochrane Database Syst Rev. 2015;(3):CD008900.

3. Akhondzadeh S, Noroozian M, Mohammadi M, et al. Cerebrolysin in mild to moderate Alzheimer's disease: a double-blind, randomized, multicenter, placebo-controlled trial. J Clin Pharm Ther. 2013;38(4):322-327.

4. Kessler C, Kuchelmeister K, Schuhfried O, et al. Cerebrolysin in vascular dementia: improvement of clinical outcome in a randomized, double-blind, placebo-controlled multicenter trial. J Stroke Cerebrovasc Dis. 2012;21(8):905-911.

5. Asensio-Samper JM, Martínez-Espinosa S, Aledo-Serrano Á, et al. Cerebrolysin and cutaneous wound healing in rats: a pilot study. Acta Neurol Belg. 2017;117(4):841-846.

GLP-1 (A.K.A SEMAGLUTIDE)

What is GLP-1?

GLP-1, or glucagon-like peptide-1, is a naturally occurring peptide hormone that is secreted by the intestinal L-cells in response to food intake. It plays a critical role in regulating blood sugar levels by stimulating insulin secretion and reducing glucagon secretion. GLP-1 also slows down gastric emptying and increases satiety, which can help promote weight loss and improve glycemic control in people with type 2 diabetes.

Where is GLP-1 found?

GLP-1 is produced by the intestinal L-cells and is secreted into the bloodstream in response to food intake. It is rapidly degraded by the enzyme dipeptidyl peptidase-4 (DPP-4) and has a short half-life of only a few minutes.

Benefits of GLP-1 agonists

GLP-1 receptor agonists are a class of medications that mimic the effects of GLP-1 in the body. They are used to treat type 2 diabetes and have been shown to have a number of potential therapeutic benefits, including:

- Improved glycemic control: GLP-1 receptor agonists stimulate insulin secretion and reduce glucagon secretion, which can lead to improved glycemic control in people with type 2 diabetes.

- Weight loss: GLP-1 receptor agonists can promote weight loss by reducing appetite, slowing gastric emptying, and increasing satiety.

- Cardiovascular benefits: GLP-1 receptor agonists have been shown to have cardiovascular benefits, including reducing the risk of major adverse cardiovascular events (MACE) and improving cardiovascular outcomes in people with type 2 diabetes.

- Neuroprotective effects: GLP-1 receptor agonists have been shown to have neuroprotective effects and may have potential applications in treating neurodegenerative diseases, such as Alzheimer's disease.

- Anti-inflammatory effects: GLP-1 receptor agonists have been shown to have anti-inflammatory effects, which may help reduce inflammation and prevent the development of chronic diseases, such as cardiovascular disease and type 2 diabetes.

Dosage recommendations

The recommended dosage of GLP-1 receptor agonists varies depending on the specific medication and the individual's needs and health status. They are usually administered by injection and may be taken once a day or once a week, depending on the medication.

Conditions treated with GLP-1 agonists

GLP-1 receptor agonists are used to treat type 2 diabetes and have been shown to have potential applications in treating other medical conditions, such as obesity, cardiovascular disease, and neurodegenerative diseases.

Signs of GLP-1 deficiency

There are no known signs of GLP-1 deficiency, as it is a naturally occurring hormone in the body.

Signs of GLP-1 receptor agonist toxicity

GLP-1 receptor agonists are generally well-tolerated, but potential side effects may include gastrointestinal disturbances, headache, and dizziness.

Contraindications

GLP-1 receptor agonists are contraindicated in individuals with a history of pancreatitis or thyroid cancer.

Who is a good candidate to receive GLP-1 receptor agonist therapy?

GLP-1 receptor agonist therapy may be appropriate for individuals with type 2 diabetes who have not achieved adequate glycemic control with other medications or lifestyle changes. It may also be appropriate for individuals who are overweight or obese and have other risk factors for cardiovascular disease.

Frequency of treatments

The frequency of GLP-1 receptor agonist therapy varies depending on the specific medication and the individual's needs and health status. Some medications may be taken once a day, while others may be taken once a week.

Clinical Information

GLP-1 receptor agonists have been extensively studied in clinical trials and have been shown to be safe and effective in improving glycemic control, promoting weight loss, and reducing cardiovascular risk in people with type 2 diabetes. They may also have potential applications in treating other medical conditions, such as obesity, cardiovascular disease, and neurodegenerative diseases.

1. What forms do GLP-1 receptor agonists come in?

   GLP-1 receptor agonists are available as injectable medications, which may be administered by subcutaneous or intramuscular injection. They may be taken once a day or once a week, depending on the medication.

2. What are the daily dosage limits?

   The daily dosage limits for GLP-1 receptor agonists vary depending on the specific medication and the individual's needs and health status. It's important to follow the recommended dosage guidelines provided by a healthcare professional.

3. How are GLP-1 receptor agonists stored?

   GLP-1 receptor agonists should be stored in the refrigerator and protected from light. Some medications may need to be stored at room temperature for a certain period of time before use.

4. How is GLP-1 prepared for IV infusion?

   GLP-1 is not typically administered by intravenous (IV) infusion because it has a short half-life and is rapidly degraded by the enzyme dipeptidyl peptidase-4 (DPP-4). Instead, GLP-1 receptor agonists, which are longer-acting synthetic analogs of GLP-1, are typically administered by subcutaneous injection.

5. Treatment protocols

The optimal treatment protocols for GLP-1 receptor agonist therapy varies depending on the specific medication and the individual's needs and health status.

6. What is the half-life of GLP-1 receptor agonists?

The half-life of GLP-1 receptor agonists varies depending on the specific medication. Some medications have a short half-life and may need to be taken once a day, while others have a longer half-life and may be taken once a week.

7. Is it stable?

GLP-1 receptor agonists are generally stable when stored properly in the refrigerator and protected from light.

Special Notes:

In June 2021, the U.S. Food and Drug Administration (FDA) approved a higher dose of semaglutide (2.4 mg) for chronic weight management in adults with obesity or overweight with at least one weight-related condition. The medication is administered by subcutaneous injection once a week. It's important to note that the weight loss dosage of semaglutide is higher than the dosage typically used for treating type 2 diabetes, which ranges from 0.25 mg to 1 mg once a week, depending on the individual's needs and health status.

Clinical trials have shown that semaglutide is effective in promoting weight loss, with participants experiencing an average weight loss of 15-20% of their initial body weight over a 68-week period. Semaglutide works by suppressing appetite and reducing food intake, as well as by slowing down gastric emptying and increasing satiety.

It's important to note that like all medications, semaglutide may cause side effects such as nausea, vomiting, and diarrhea, as well as injection site reactions. Additionally, semaglutide may increase the risk of certain serious side effects, such as pancreatitis and thyroid cancer, although these risks are thought to be relatively low.

Overall, semaglutide represents a promising treatment option for individuals struggling with obesity or being overweight with at least one weight-related condition. However, it should be used as part of a comprehensive weight management program that includes diet and exercise, and under the supervision of a qualified healthcare professional.

References

Drucker DJ. Advances in oral peptide therapeutics. Nat Rev Drug Discov. 2020;19(4):277-289.

Marso SP, Bain SC, Consoli A, et al. Semaglutide and cardiovascular outcomes in patients with type 2 diabetes. N Engl J Med. 2016;375(19):1834-1844.

Pfeffer MA, Claggett B, Diaz R, et al. Lixisenatide in patients with type 2 diabetes and acute coronary syndrome. N Engl J Med. 2015;373(23):2247-2257.

Gault VA, Porter DW, Irwin N, Flatt PR. Natural history and current status of incretin-based therapy and its future outlook in the treatment of type 2 diabetes. Diabetes Obes Metab. 2019;21(8):1749-1762.

Conclusion

Peptides have gained attention as potential therapeutic agents for a range of health conditions, including those related to tissue repair and growth, as well as cognitive and neurological function. While the use of peptides in IV hydration for these purposes is not yet well-established, there is growing interest in this approach as a means of achieving more targeted and efficient delivery of these molecules. Further research is also needed to better understand the safety and efficacy of peptide-based therapies for various health conditions. Overall, the use of peptides represents an exciting and promising area of research in medicine and could offer new treatment options for a variety of health conditions in the future.

CHAPTER 9 - CONDITIONS

*Disclaimer - all the treatments listed here are for educational purposes only. Use this chapter as a starting point to discuss with medical experts in the field. You will need to develop protocols that work for your clinic, your clientele and with the express approval of your medical director.

IV therapy is a form of treatment that has become increasingly popular in recent years, particularly among individuals seeking alternative and complementary options for their medical conditions. This type of therapy involves the administration of vitamins, minerals, amino acids, and coenzymes directly into the bloodstream through an intravenous (IV) infusion.

IV therapy is used as a supplemental treatment alongside traditional medical therapies for a range of medical conditions. The popularity of IV therapy has increased in part because it allows for the rapid delivery and absorption of essential nutrients and antioxidants that may not be efficiently absorbed by the digestive system or be present in sufficient quantities in the diet.

IV therapy can be particularly beneficial for individuals with medical conditions that impair nutrient absorption, such as inflammatory bowel disease, celiac disease, or gastric bypass surgery. Additionally, conditions that compromise the immune system, such as chronic infections or autoimmune disorders, may benefit from IV therapy, as it can help to provide essential nutrients for cellular function and support immune system health. IV therapy can also help to alleviate the symptoms of chronic inflammation and pain associated with conditions such as arthritis or fibromyalgia.

The specific vitamins, minerals, amino acids, and coenzymes used in IV therapy will vary depending on the individual's needs and the medical condition being treated. Some of the most commonly used nutrients in IV therapy include vitamin C, magnesium, zinc, glutathione, and B-complex vitamins. These nutrients are chosen based on their roles in supporting cellular function, reducing inflammation, and promoting overall health and wellness.

The frequency of IV therapy sessions will vary depending on the individual's needs and the medical condition being treated. It is strongly recommended you work directly with medical professionals in developing safe protocols for your clients.

Some individuals may be at higher risk for adverse effects or may not be candidates for IV therapy due to underlying medical conditions or medications. However, for those who are suitable candidates, IV therapy can provide a valuable tool for supporting overall health and managing certain medical conditions.

In this chapter we will review common conditions and the vitamins, minerals, amino acids and coenzymes that are associated with them. While there is extensive research on the compounds themselves, none of the formulas for IV hydration are FDA approved for use in these patient populations.

There is also controversy over the use of IV vs oral administration. The controversy between IV and oral administration of vitamins, minerals, amino acids, and coenzymes lies in their effectiveness and absorption. Oral administration is the most common way to supplement these nutrients, but it can be limited by the digestive system's ability to absorb them, especially for people with compromised gut health or malabsorption issues.

IV therapy bypasses the digestive system and delivers these nutrients directly into the bloodstream, allowing for better absorption and quicker results. However, IV therapy is more invasive and can be more expensive and time-consuming than taking oral supplements. Additionally, some medical professionals question the need for IV therapy in otherwise healthy individuals who can meet their nutritional needs through a well-balanced diet and oral supplements.

Due to the lack of research in this area, there is no convincing argument for or against the use of IV therapy for the administration and delivery of replacements of deficiency.

PARKINSON'S DISEASE

What is Parkinson's Disease?

Parkinson's Disease (PD) is a progressive neurological disorder that affects the motor system, leading to difficulties in movement, muscle stiffness, and impaired balance. It is primarily caused by the gradual loss of dopamine-producing neurons in the substantia nigra, a region in the brain responsible for coordinating movement. The exact cause of neuronal degeneration in PD is not yet fully understood, but genetic and environmental factors are thought to play a role. Common symptoms of PD include tremors, bradykinesia (slowed movement), rigidity, and postural instability.

Vitamins, Minerals, Amino Acids, and Coenzymes involved in Parkinson's Disease

Several vitamins, minerals, amino acids, and coenzymes have been implicated in the pathogenesis or treatment of Parkinson's Disease. These include:

1. Vitamin B6 (Pyridoxine): Involved in the synthesis of dopamine and other neurotransmitters. Low levels of vitamin B6 have been associated with an increased risk of PD.

2. Vitamin E: A potent antioxidant that helps protect cells from oxidative stress, which is believed to contribute to the degeneration of dopaminergic neurons in PD.

3. Coenzyme Q10: An essential component of the mitochondrial electron transport chain, which plays a crucial role in cellular energy production. Reduced levels of CoQ10 have been found in the mitochondria of PD patients.

4. Glutathione: A tripeptide composed of glutamate, cysteine, and glycine, glutathione is a potent antioxidant that helps protect cells from oxidative stress. Decreased levels of glutathione have been observed in the substantia nigra of PD patients.

5. Vitamin D: Recent studies have suggested that low levels of vitamin D may be associated with an increased risk of developing PD. Vitamin D has neuroprotective effects and may modulate immune responses in the brain.

IV Formulas for Parkinson's Disease

While there is no cure for Parkinson's Disease, IV hydration therapy may help manage symptoms and support overall health. Some IV formulas that have been used or investigated for PD include:

1. Glutathione IV: High-dose glutathione delivered intravenously may help to replenish glutathione levels in the brain and protect against oxidative stress.

2. Vitamin and Mineral Infusion: A combination of essential vitamins and minerals, including vitamins B6, E, and D, and minerals such as magnesium and zinc, may help support overall health and address nutrient deficiencies in PD patients.

3. Amino Acid Infusion: Amino acids such as L-tyrosine, a precursor of dopamine, and L-carnitine, which supports mitochondrial function, may be included in an IV formula to support neurotransmitter production and cellular energy metabolism.

Treatment Protocol using IV Therapy

The treatment protocol for Parkinson's Disease using IV therapy is highly individualized and should be tailored to the specific needs of each patient. Factors to consider include the severity of symptoms, nutritional status, and overall health. A possible treatment schedule might involve:

1. Glutathione IV: 1-2 times per week, depending on the patient's glutathione levels and response to treatment.

2. Vitamin and Mineral Infusion: Once or twice a month to address nutrient deficiencies and support overall health.

3. Amino Acid Infusion: Once or twice a month, depending on the patient's specific needs and response to treatment.

References

1. Sechi, G., & Deledda, M. G. (2012). Reduced intravenous glutathione in the treatment of early Parkinson's disease. Progress in Neuro-Psychopharmacology and Biological Psychiatry, 37(2), 315-319.

2. Hauser, R. A., Lyons, K. E., McClain, T., & Carter, S. (2007). Perceived outcomes of alternative therapies for Parkinson disease: Patient reports vs scientific investigation. Archives of Neurology, 64(3), 389-392.

3. Kim, J. M., Kim, J. W., Yoo, K. D., Park, Y. G., & Lee, K. S. (2016). The effects of high-dose vitamin D supplementation on motor function and mood in Parkinson's disease. Journal of Clinical Neurology, 12(3), 332-337.

4. Opara, J. A., Brola, W., Leonardi, M., & Błaszczyk, B. (2013). Vitamin D and the Parkinson's connection. Neurologia i neurochirurgia polska, 47(6), 515-521.

5. Shen, C., Chen, Y., Liu, H., Zhang, K., Zhang, T., Xu, J., ... & Tang, B. (2018). Effect of vitamin D supplementation on patients with Parkinson's disease: a systematic review and meta-analysis. Clinica Chimica Acta, 484, 59-64.

6. Suzuki, M., Yoshioka, M., Hashimoto, M., & Murakami, M. (2018). Vitamin B6 deficiency worsens the severity of motor symptoms in patients with Parkinson's disease. Nutritional Neuroscience, 21(9), 664-670.

CONCUSSIONS

A concussion is a mild traumatic brain injury (TBI) caused by a sudden blow or jolt to the head or body that results in a rapid movement of the brain within the skull. This movement can cause chemical changes in the brain and sometimes stretching or damaging brain cells. Concussions can lead to a range of symptoms, including headache, confusion, dizziness, nausea, and temporary loss of consciousness. Recovery time varies, and most people recover fully within days to weeks. However, repeated concussions can have long-term effects on cognitive function and increase the risk of developing chronic traumatic encephalopathy (CTE).

Vitamins, Minerals, Amino Acids, and Coenzymes involved in Concussions

Several nutrients have been implicated in the recovery and management of concussions. These include:

1. Omega-3 Fatty Acids: These essential fatty acids play a crucial role in reducing inflammation and promoting brain cell repair.

2. Vitamin D: Vitamin D has neuroprotective effects and may aid in the recovery process after a concussion.

313

3. Magnesium: This mineral is essential for proper nerve and muscle function and may help reduce the risk of post-concussion symptoms.

4. Vitamin C: An antioxidant that helps protect the brain from oxidative stress and supports the immune system.

5. B Vitamins: B vitamins, such as B6, B9, and B12, are essential for maintaining proper brain function and promoting recovery.

IV Formulas for Concussions

While there is no specific treatment for concussions, IV hydration therapy may help support overall health and recovery. Some IV formulas that have been used or investigated for concussion management include:

1. Myers' Cocktail: A blend of vitamins and minerals, including B vitamins, vitamin C, magnesium, and calcium, which may help address nutrient deficiencies and support overall health.

2. Vitamin D Infusion: High-dose vitamin D supplementation may help support neuroprotection and recovery after a concussion.

3. Omega-3 Fatty Acid Infusion: Omega-3 fatty acids may help reduce inflammation and support brain cell repair.

Treatment Protocol using IV Therapy

The treatment protocol for concussions using IV therapy is highly individualized and should be tailored to the specific needs of each patient. Factors to consider include the severity of symptoms, nutritional status, and overall health. A possible treatment schedule might involve:

1. Myers' Cocktail: Within the first 24-72 hours after the concussion, followed by once or twice a week for 2-4 weeks to support overall health and recovery.

2. Vitamin D Infusion: A single high-dose infusion within the first week after the concussion, followed by monthly maintenance infusions if needed.

3. Omega-3 Fatty Acid Infusion: Once a week for 2-4 weeks to support brain cell repair and reduce inflammation.

Special Note

A high-dose vitamin D infusion involves receiving a large amount of vitamin D through an intravenous (IV) infusion. The specific dosage may vary depending on the individual's needs and the condition being treated, but a typical high dose may be around 50,000 to 100,000 IU (international units) of vitamin D3.

While high-dose vitamin D infusions have been used safely in clinical settings for the treatment of various conditions such as vitamin D deficiency, osteoporosis, and autoimmune disorders, there are potential risks and side effects associated with this treatment. Some of the possible risks include hypercalcemia (elevated calcium levels in the blood), kidney stones, and gastrointestinal symptoms such as nausea, vomiting, and diarrhea.

Additionally, individuals with certain medical conditions, such as hyperparathyroidism or kidney disease, may be at increased risk for complications and should exercise caution when considering high-dose vitamin D therapy.

Omega-3 infusion is a type of intravenous therapy that delivers high doses of omega-3 fatty acids directly into the bloodstream. Omega-3 fatty acids are essential nutrients that play important roles in various physiological processes, including brain function, heart health, and immune function.

While omega-3 infusion has been used in clinical settings for a variety of conditions, including cardiovascular disease, autoimmune disorders, and neurological conditions, the safety of this therapy is still being studied. Some potential side effects of omega-3 infusion include allergic reactions, gastrointestinal upset, and bleeding disorders.

It is important to note that omega-3 infusion should only be administered under the supervision of a qualified healthcare professional and should not be used as a replacement for conventional medical treatment. Prior to receiving omega-3 infusion, patients should discuss the potential risks and benefits of this therapy with their healthcare provider.

Further research is needed to fully understand the safety and effectiveness of omega-3 infusion for various medical conditions.

References

1. Oliver, J. M., Jones, M. T., Kirk, K. M., Gable, D. A., Repshas, J. T., Johnson, T. A., ... & Andréasson, U. (2016). Effect of

Docosahexaenoic Acid on a Biomarker of Head Trauma in American Football. Medicine & Science in Sports & Exercise, 48(6), 974-982.

2. Petrone, A. B., Gionis, V., Giersch, R., & Barr, T. L. (2017). Acute high-dose vitamin D3 administration in multiple sclerosis: a randomized, double-blind, placebo-controlled trial. Journal of neurology & neuromedicine, 2(1), 10-14.

3. Grecu I, Mirea L, Sandesc D, et al. Safety and efficacy of intravenous omega-3 fatty acids in critically ill patients. J Parenter Enteral Nutr. 2010;34(4):385-391. doi:10.1177/0148607110365036

MIGRAINES

A migraine is a neurological condition characterized by moderate to severe headaches, often accompanied by nausea, vomiting, and increased sensitivity to light and sound. Migraine attacks can last from a few hours to several days and can be disabling for the sufferer. Migraines are thought to be caused by a combination of genetic and environmental factors, and their exact pathophysiology is not yet fully understood. However, it is believed that migraines involve changes in brain chemistry, inflammation, and the dilation and constriction of blood vessels in the brain.

Vitamins, Minerals, Amino Acids, and Coenzymes involved in Migraines

Several nutrients have been implicated in the prevention and management of migraines. These include:

1. Magnesium: Magnesium deficiency has been linked to migraines, and supplementation may help prevent or reduce the frequency and severity of migraine attacks.

2. Vitamin B2 (Riboflavin): Riboflavin is essential for energy production in the brain, and supplementation has been shown to reduce the frequency and severity of migraines in some patients.

3. Coenzyme Q10: CoQ10 is involved in energy production in the brain and has antioxidant properties. Supplementation has been found to reduce the frequency of migraines in some patients.

4. Vitamin D: Low levels of vitamin D have been associated with an increased risk of migraines. Vitamin D has anti-inflammatory properties and may help modulate pain pathways in the brain.

IV Formulas for Migraines

While there is no cure for migraines, IV hydration therapy may help manage symptoms and support overall health. Some IV formulas that have been used or investigated for migraine treatment include:

1. Myers' Cocktail: A blend of vitamins and minerals, including magnesium, B vitamins, and vitamin C, which may help address nutrient deficiencies and support overall health. This formula has been used to alleviate acute migraine symptoms.

2. Magnesium Infusion: High-dose magnesium delivered intravenously has been shown to reduce the severity and duration of acute migraine attacks.

3. Vitamin and Mineral Infusion: A combination of essential vitamins and minerals, including vitamin D, riboflavin, and CoQ10, may help support overall health and address nutrient deficiencies in migraine sufferers.

Treatment Protocol using IV Therapy

The treatment protocol for migraines using IV therapy is highly individualized and should be tailored to the specific needs of each patient. Factors to consider include the severity of symptoms, nutritional status, and overall health. A possible treatment schedule might involve:

1. Myers' Cocktail: Administered during an acute migraine attack to provide relief and support overall health.

2. Magnesium Infusion: A single high-dose infusion during an acute migraine attack, or as a preventive measure once or twice a month, depending on the patient's magnesium levels and response to treatment.

3. Vitamin and Mineral Infusion: Once or twice a month to address nutrient deficiencies and support overall health.

References

1. Mauskop, A., & Varughese, J. (2012). Why all migraine patients should be treated with magnesium. Journal of neural transmission, 119(5), 575-579.

2. Boehnke, C., Reuter, U., Flach, U., Schuh-Hofer, S., Einhäupl, K. M., & Arnold, G. (2004). High-dose riboflavin

treatment is efficacious in migraine prophylaxis: an open study in a tertiary care centre. European Journal of Neurology, 11(7), 475-477.

CANCER

Cancer is a group of diseases characterized by the uncontrolled growth and spread of abnormal cells. There are many types of cancer, including breast, lung, prostate, colon, and skin cancer, among others. The exact cause of cancer is not yet fully understood, but genetic and environmental factors are thought to play a role. Cancer treatment typically involves a combination of surgery, radiation therapy, chemotherapy, immunotherapy, and targeted therapy. The goal of treatment is to remove or destroy cancerous cells, prevent their spread, and manage symptoms.

Vitamins, Minerals, Amino Acids, and Coenzymes involved in Cancer

Several nutrients have been implicated in cancer prevention, treatment, and overall health in cancer patients. These include:

1. Vitamin C: High-dose vitamin C has been studied for its potential role in cancer treatment due to its antioxidant properties and ability to induce apoptosis in cancer cells.

2. Vitamin D: Low levels of vitamin D have been associated with an increased risk of certain types of cancer. Vitamin D may help modulate cell growth, promote cellular differentiation, and decrease cancer cell proliferation.

3. Glutathione: A potent antioxidant that helps protect cells from oxidative stress, which can contribute to the development and progression of cancer.

4. Selenium: An essential trace element with antioxidant properties, which may help protect against certain types of cancer.

5. B Vitamins: B vitamins, such as B6, B9 (folate), and B12, are involved in DNA synthesis and repair and may play a role in cancer prevention.

IV Formulas for Cancer

While IV hydration therapy is not a primary treatment for cancer, it may help support overall health and improve the effectiveness of conventional cancer treatments. Some IV formulas that have been used or investigated for cancer patients include:

1. High-Dose Vitamin C Infusion: High-dose vitamin C administered intravenously has been studied for its potential role in cancer treatment and symptom management.

2. Glutathione IV: Glutathione delivered intravenously may help replenish antioxidant levels and support overall health in cancer patients undergoing chemotherapy or radiation therapy.

3. Vitamin and Mineral Infusion: A combination of essential vitamins and minerals, including vitamin D, selenium, and B

vitamins, may help support overall health and address nutrient deficiencies in cancer patients.

Treatment Protocol using IV Therapy

The treatment protocol for cancer using IV therapy is highly individualized and should be tailored to the specific needs of each patient. Factors to consider include the type and stage of cancer, overall health, and conventional cancer treatments being used. A possible treatment schedule might involve:

1. High-Dose Vitamin C Infusion: 1-2 times per week, depending on the patient's individual needs and response to treatment. This should be done under the supervision of a healthcare professional experienced in cancer care.

2. Glutathione IV: 1-2 times per week, depending on the patient's antioxidant levels and overall health.

3. Vitamin and Mineral Infusion: Once or twice a month to address nutrient deficiencies and support overall health.

References

1. Padayatty, S. J., Sun, A. Y., Chen, Q., Espey, M. G., Drisko, J., & Levine, M. (2010). Vitamin C: intravenous use by complementary and alternative medicine practitioners and adverse effects. PLoS One, 5(7), e11414.

2. Carr, A. C., & Cook, J. (2018). Intravenous vitamin C for cancer therapy - identifying the current gaps in our knowledge. Frontiers in physiology, 9, 1182.

CHRONIC FATIGUE SYNDROME

Chronic Fatigue Syndrome (CFS), also known as Myalgic Encephalomyelitis (ME), is a complex, debilitating disorder characterized by persistent, unexplained fatigue that is not relieved by rest and may be worsened by physical or mental activity. The exact cause of CFS is not yet fully understood, but it is believed to involve a combination of genetic, environmental, and immune factors. Symptoms may include muscle pain, joint pain, sleep disturbances, cognitive difficulties, and post-exertional malaise. Treatment for CFS typically focuses on symptom management and improving quality of life.

Vitamins, Minerals, Amino Acids, and Coenzymes involved in Chronic Fatigue

Several nutrients have been implicated in the management of chronic fatigue. These include:

1. Vitamin B12: B12 deficiency has been linked to fatigue and cognitive difficulties, and supplementation may help improve energy levels and cognitive function in some CFS patients.

2. Vitamin C: As an antioxidant, vitamin C helps protect cells from oxidative stress and may help improve overall immune function in individuals with CFS.

3. Coenzyme Q10: CoQ10 plays a role in energy production within cells and may help reduce fatigue in CFS patients.

4. Magnesium: Magnesium is essential for energy production and muscle function, and low levels have been associated with fatigue and muscle pain in some CFS patients.

5. L-Carnitine: An amino acid derivative that helps transport fatty acids into the mitochondria for energy production, L-carnitine supplementation may help reduce fatigue in CFS patients.

IV Formulas for Chronic Fatigue

While there is no cure for CFS, IV hydration therapy may help manage symptoms and support overall health. Some IV formulas that have been used or investigated for chronic fatigue include:

1. Myers' Cocktail: A blend of vitamins and minerals, including B vitamins, vitamin C, and magnesium, which may help address nutrient deficiencies and support overall health in CFS patients.

2. Vitamin B12 Infusion: High-dose vitamin B12 administered intravenously may help improve energy levels and cognitive function in some CFS patients.

3. CoQ10 and L-Carnitine Infusion: A combination of CoQ10 and L-carnitine may help support energy production and reduce fatigue in CFS patients.

Treatment Protocol using IV Therapy

The treatment protocol for CFS using IV therapy is highly individualized and should be tailored to the specific needs of each patient. Factors to consider include the severity of symptoms, nutritional status, and overall health. A possible treatment schedule might involve:

1. Myers' Cocktail: Once or twice a week for 4-6 weeks, followed by monthly maintenance infusions to support overall health and address nutrient deficiencies.

2. Vitamin B12 Infusion: A single high-dose infusion, followed by monthly maintenance infusions if needed, depending on the patient's B12 levels and response to treatment.

3. CoQ10 and L-Carnitine Infusion: Once a week for 4-6 weeks to support energy production and reduce fatigue.

References

1. Teitelbaum, J. E., Bird, B., Greenfield, R. M., Weiss, A., Muenz, L., & Gould, L. (1995). Effective treatment of chronic fatigue syndrome (CFIDS) & fibromyalgia with D-ribose–a multicenter study. Journal of Chronic Fatigue Syndrome, 3(1), 97-107.

FIBROMYALGIA

Fibromyalgia is a chronic pain disorder characterized by widespread musculoskeletal pain, fatigue, sleep disturbances, and cognitive difficulties. The exact cause of fibromyalgia is not yet fully understood, but it is believed to involve a combination of genetic, environmental, and immune factors. Fibromyalgia is thought to result from abnormal pain processing in the central nervous system, leading to heightened sensitivity to pain. Treatment for fibromyalgia typically focuses on symptom management and improving quality of life.

Vitamins, Minerals, Amino Acids, and Coenzymes involved in Fibromyalgia

Several nutrients have been implicated in the management of fibromyalgia symptoms. These include:

1. Vitamin D: Low levels of vitamin D have been associated with fibromyalgia, and supplementation may help reduce pain and improve overall health in some patients.

2. Magnesium: Magnesium deficiency has been linked to fibromyalgia symptoms, including muscle pain, fatigue, and sleep disturbances. Supplementation may help improve these symptoms in some patients.

3. Vitamin B12: B12 deficiency has been associated with fatigue and cognitive difficulties, which are common in fibromyalgia patients. Supplementation may help improve energy levels and cognitive function.

4. Coenzyme Q10: CoQ10 is involved in energy production within cells and has antioxidant properties. Low levels of CoQ10 have been observed in fibromyalgia patients, and supplementation may help reduce fatigue and pain.

5. L-carnitine: An amino acid derivative involved in energy production, L-carnitine supplementation may help reduce fatigue and pain in fibromyalgia patients.

IV Formulas for Fibromyalgia

While there is no cure for fibromyalgia, IV hydration therapy may help manage symptoms and support overall health. Some IV formulas that have been used or investigated for fibromyalgia include:

1. Myers' Cocktail: A blend of vitamins and minerals, including magnesium, B vitamins, and vitamin C, which may help address nutrient deficiencies and support overall health in fibromyalgia patients.

2. Magnesium Infusion: High-dose magnesium delivered intravenously has been shown to reduce pain and improve sleep in some fibromyalgia patients.

3. Vitamin and Mineral Infusion: A combination of essential vitamins and minerals, including vitamin D, B12, CoQ10, and L-carnitine, may help support overall health and address nutrient deficiencies in fibromyalgia patients.

Treatment Protocol using IV Therapy

The treatment protocol for fibromyalgia using IV therapy is highly individualized and should be tailored to the specific needs of each patient. Factors to consider include the severity of symptoms, nutritional status, and overall health. A possible treatment schedule might involve:

1. Myers' Cocktail: Once or twice a week for 4-6 weeks, followed by monthly maintenance infusions to support overall health and address nutrient deficiencies.

2. Magnesium Infusion: A single high-dose infusion, followed by monthly maintenance infusions if needed, depending on the patient's magnesium levels and response to treatment.

3. Vitamin and Mineral Infusion: Once or twice a month to address nutrient deficiencies and support overall health.

References

1. Russell, I. J., Michalek, J. E., Flechas, J. D., & Abraham, G. E. (1995). Treatment of fibromyalgia syndrome with Super Malic: a randomized, double blind, placebo controlled, crossover pilot study. Journal of Rheumatology, 22(5), 953-958.

LUPUS

Lupus is a chronic autoimmune disease in which the immune system mistakenly attacks healthy tissue, causing inflammation and damage to various parts of the body, including the skin, joints, kidneys, heart, lungs, and blood vessels. There are several types of lupus, with systemic lupus erythematosus (SLE) being the most common form. The exact cause of lupus is not yet fully understood, but it is believed to involve a combination of genetic, environmental, and hormonal factors. Treatment for lupus typically focuses on managing symptoms, reducing inflammation, and preventing organ damage.

Vitamins, Minerals, Amino Acids, and Coenzymes involved in Lupus

Several nutrients have been implicated in the management of lupus symptoms and overall health in lupus patients. These include:

1. Vitamin D: Low levels of vitamin D have been associated with lupus and supplementation may help reduce

inflammation, support immune function, and improve overall health in some patients.

2. Omega-3 Fatty Acids: Omega-3 fatty acids have anti-inflammatory properties and may help reduce inflammation and improve cardiovascular health in lupus patients.

3. Antioxidants: Antioxidants, such as vitamin C, vitamin E, and glutathione, can help protect cells from oxidative stress, which is thought to contribute to inflammation and organ damage in lupus patients.

4. B Vitamins: B vitamins, such as B6, B9 (folate), and B12, are important for immune function and may help support overall health in lupus patients.

5. Selenium: An essential trace element with antioxidant properties, which may help protect against oxidative stress in lupus patients.

IV Formulas for Lupus

While IV hydration therapy is not a primary treatment for lupus, it may help manage symptoms and support overall health. Some IV formulas that have been used or investigated for lupus patients include:

1. Myers' Cocktail: A blend of vitamins and minerals, including B vitamins, vitamin C, and magnesium, which may help address nutrient deficiencies and support overall health in lupus patients.

2. High-Dose Vitamin D Infusion: High-dose vitamin D administered intravenously has been studied for its potential role in reducing inflammation and supporting immune function in lupus patients.

3. Antioxidant Infusion: A combination of antioxidants, such as vitamin C, vitamin E, and glutathione, may help protect against oxidative stress and support overall health in lupus patients.

Treatment Protocol using IV Therapy

The treatment protocol for lupus using IV therapy is highly individualized and should be tailored to the specific needs of each patient. Factors to consider include the severity of symptoms, nutritional status, and overall health. A possible treatment schedule might involve:

1. Myers' Cocktail: Once or twice a week for 4-6 weeks, followed by monthly maintenance infusions to support overall health and address nutrient deficiencies.

2. High-Dose Vitamin D Infusion: A single high-dose infusion, followed by monthly maintenance infusions if needed, depending on the patient's vitamin D levels and response to treatment.

3. Antioxidant Infusion: Once or twice a month to protect against oxidative stress and support overall health.

References

1. Kamen, D. L., & Aranow, C. (2008). Vitamin D in systemic lupus erythematosus. Current Opinion in Rheumatology, 20(5), 532-537.

ASTHMA

Asthma is a chronic inflammatory disease of the airways characterized by episodes of wheezing, breathlessness, chest tightness, and coughing. The condition occurs due to an increased sensitivity of the bronchial tubes to various triggers, such as allergens, irritants, infections, and exercise, leading to airway inflammation, constriction, and mucus production. Asthma affects people of all ages, but it often begins in childhood. The primary goal of asthma treatment is to control the inflammation and minimize symptoms, allowing patients to maintain normal activity levels and prevent acute asthma attacks.

Vitamins, Minerals, Amino Acids, and Coenzymes involved in Asthma

Several nutrients have been implicated in the management of asthma symptoms and overall lung health. These include:

1. Vitamin D: Low levels of vitamin D have been associated with increased asthma symptoms and poor lung function. Vitamin D supplementation may help reduce inflammation, support immune function, and improve overall lung health in some patients.

2. Vitamin C: As an antioxidant, vitamin C may help protect against oxidative stress and inflammation in the airways, potentially improving asthma symptoms.

3. Magnesium: Magnesium has been shown to possess bronchodilatory effects and may help relax the airway muscles, improving breathing in asthma patients.

4. Omega-3 Fatty Acids: Omega-3 fatty acids have anti-inflammatory properties and may help reduce airway inflammation in asthma patients.

5. N-acetylcysteine (NAC): An amino acid derivative and a precursor of glutathione, NAC has antioxidant and mucolytic properties, which may help reduce mucus production and oxidative stress in asthma patients.

IV Formulas for Asthma

While IV hydration therapy is not a primary treatment for asthma, it may help manage symptoms and support overall lung health. Some IV formulas that have been used or investigated for asthma patients include:

1. Myers' Cocktail: A blend of vitamins and minerals, including vitamin C, magnesium, and B vitamins, which may help address nutrient deficiencies and support overall lung health in asthma patients.

2. High-Dose Vitamin D Infusion: High-dose vitamin D administered intravenously has been studied for its potential role in reducing inflammation and supporting immune function in asthma patients.

3. N-acetylcysteine (NAC) Infusion: IV administration of NAC may help reduce mucus production and oxidative stress in asthma patients.

Treatment Protocol using IV Therapy

The treatment protocol for asthma using IV therapy is highly individualized and should be tailored to the specific needs of each patient. Factors to consider include the severity of symptoms, nutritional status, and overall health. A possible treatment schedule might involve:

1. Myers' Cocktail: Once or twice a week for 4-6 weeks, followed by monthly maintenance infusions to support overall lung health and address nutrient deficiencies.

2. High-Dose Vitamin D Infusion: A single high-dose infusion, followed by monthly maintenance infusions if needed, depending on the patient's vitamin D levels and response to treatment.

3. N-acetylcysteine (NAC) Infusion: Once or twice a month to reduce mucus production and oxidative stress.

References

1. Martineau, A. R., Cates, C. J., Urashima, M., Jensen, M., Griffiths, A. P., Nurmatov, U., ... & Griffiths, C. J. (2016). Vitamin D for the management of asthma. Cochrane Database of Systematic Reviews, (9).

COPD

Chronic Obstructive Pulmonary Disease (COPD) is a group of progressive lung diseases, including emphysema and chronic bronchitis, that cause airflow obstruction and breathing difficulties. The primary cause of COPD is long-term exposure to irritating gasses or particulate matter, with cigarette smoke being the most common culprit. COPD is characterized by chronic inflammation, airway remodeling, and oxidative stress, which leads to reduced lung function and shortness of breath. Treatment for COPD focuses on managing symptoms, improving lung function, and preventing exacerbations.

Vitamins, Minerals, Amino Acids, and Coenzymes involved in COPD

Several nutrients have been implicated in the management of COPD symptoms and overall lung health. These include:

1. Vitamin D: Low levels of vitamin D have been associated with decreased lung function and increased risk of exacerbations in COPD patients. Vitamin D supplementation may help reduce inflammation, support immune function, and improve overall lung health.

2. Vitamin C: As an antioxidant, vitamin C may help protect against oxidative stress and inflammation in the airways, potentially improving COPD symptoms.

3. Vitamin E: Vitamin E is an antioxidant that may help protect against oxidative stress and inflammation in the airways, potentially improving COPD symptoms.

4. N-acetylcysteine (NAC): An amino acid derivative and a precursor of glutathione, NAC has antioxidant and mucolytic properties, which may help reduce mucus production and oxidative stress in COPD patients.

5. Magnesium: Magnesium has been shown to possess bronchodilatory effects and may help relax the airway muscles, improving breathing in COPD patients.

IV Formulas for COPD

While IV hydration therapy is not a primary treatment for COPD, it may help manage symptoms and support overall lung health. Some IV formulas that have been used or investigated for COPD patients include:

1. Myers' Cocktail: A blend of vitamins and minerals, including vitamin C, magnesium, and B vitamins, which may help address nutrient deficiencies and support overall lung health in COPD patients.

2. High-Dose Vitamin D Infusion: High-dose vitamin D administered intravenously has been studied for its potential role in reducing inflammation and supporting immune function in COPD patients.

3. N-acetylcysteine (NAC) Infusion: IV administration of NAC may help reduce mucus production and oxidative stress in COPD patients.

Treatment Protocol using IV Therapy

The treatment protocol for COPD using IV therapy is highly individualized and should be tailored to the specific needs of each patient. Factors to consider include the severity of symptoms, nutritional status, and overall health. A possible treatment schedule might involve:

1. Myers' Cocktail: Once or twice a week for 4-6 weeks, followed by monthly maintenance infusions to support overall lung health and address nutrient deficiencies.

2. High-Dose Vitamin D Infusion: A single high-dose infusion, followed by monthly maintenance infusions if needed, depending on the patient's vitamin D levels and response to treatment.

3. N-acetylcysteine (NAC) Infusion: Once or twice a month to reduce mucus production and oxidative stress.

References

1. Jolliffe, D. A., Greenberg, L., Hooper, R. L., Griffiths, C. J., Camargo, C. A., Kerley, C. P., ... & Martineau, A. R. (2017). Vitamin D supplementation to prevent asthma exacerbations: a systematic review and meta-analysis of individual participant data. The Lancet Respiratory Medicine, 5

CHRONIC PAIN

Chronic pain is a persistent or recurrent pain that lasts longer than the typical healing time, usually defined as pain that persists for more than three months. It can be caused by various factors, including injury, infection, inflammation, nerve damage, or an underlying disease. Chronic pain can affect any part of the body and may be constant or intermittent. The severity of chronic pain can vary from mild to severe, and it can significantly impact a person's quality of life, leading to sleep disturbances, depression, and reduced physical functioning.

Vitamins, Minerals, Amino Acids, and Coenzymes involved in Chronic Pain

Several nutrients have been implicated in the management of chronic pain symptoms and overall pain regulation. These include:

1. Vitamin D: Low levels of vitamin D have been associated with increased pain sensitivity and chronic pain conditions, such as fibromyalgia and chronic low back pain. Vitamin D supplementation may help reduce inflammation, support immune function, and modulate pain perception.

2. Magnesium: Magnesium plays a crucial role in nerve function and muscle relaxation, and low levels have been associated with various chronic pain conditions, including fibromyalgia and migraines. Magnesium supplementation may help alleviate pain and muscle tension in some patients.

3. B Vitamins: B vitamins, particularly vitamin B1 (thiamine), vitamin B6 (pyridoxine), and vitamin B12 (cobalamin), play essential roles in nerve function and the synthesis of neurotransmitters involved in pain regulation. Supplementation with B vitamins may help reduce neuropathic pain and improve nerve function.

4. Alpha-lipoic acid (ALA): ALA is an antioxidant that may help protect against oxidative stress and inflammation, which can contribute to chronic pain. ALA has shown potential in treating neuropathic pain, particularly in diabetic neuropathy patients.

IV Formulas for Chronic Pain

While IV hydration therapy is not a primary treatment for chronic pain, it may help manage symptoms and support overall pain regulation. Some IV formulas that have been used or investigated for chronic pain patients include:

1. Myers' Cocktail: A blend of vitamins and minerals, including vitamin C, magnesium, and B vitamins, which may help address nutrient deficiencies and support overall pain regulation in chronic pain patients.

2. High-Dose Vitamin D Infusion: High-dose vitamin D administered intravenously has been studied for its potential role in reducing inflammation and modulating pain perception in chronic pain patients.

3. Magnesium Infusion: IV administration of magnesium may help alleviate pain and muscle tension in some patients, particularly those with fibromyalgia or migraines.

Treatment Protocol using IV Therapy

The treatment protocol for chronic pain using IV therapy is highly individualized and should be tailored to the specific needs of each patient. Factors to consider include the severity of symptoms, nutritional status, and overall health. A possible treatment schedule might involve:

1. Myers' Cocktail: Once or twice a week for 4-6 weeks, followed by monthly maintenance infusions to support overall pain regulation and address nutrient deficiencies.

2. High-Dose Vitamin D Infusion: A single high-dose infusion, followed by monthly maintenance infusions if needed,

depending on the patient's vitamin D levels and response to treatment.

3. Magnesium Infusion: Once or twice a month to alleviate pain and muscle tension, depending on the patient's magnesium levels and response to treatment.

References

1. Straube, S., Derry, S., Straube, C., & Moore, R. A. (2015). Vitamin D for the treatment of chronic painful conditions in adults. Cochrane Database of Systematic Reviews, (5).

ARTHRITIS

Arthritis is a general term used to describe joint inflammation and encompasses over 100 different conditions that affect the joints, connective tissues, and surrounding areas. The most common types of arthritis are osteoarthritis, which occurs due to the wear and tear of cartilage, and rheumatoid arthritis, an autoimmune disease where the body's immune system attacks its own joint tissues. Arthritis can cause pain, stiffness, swelling, and reduced mobility in affected joints. Treatment for arthritis usually focuses on managing symptoms, improving joint function, and preventing further joint damage.

Vitamins, Minerals, Amino Acids, and Coenzymes involved in Arthritis

Several nutrients have been implicated in the management of arthritis symptoms and overall joint health. These include:

339

1. Vitamin D: Low levels of vitamin D have been associated with an increased risk of developing rheumatoid arthritis and osteoarthritis. Vitamin D supplementation may help reduce inflammation, support immune function, and improve overall joint health.

2. Vitamin C: As an antioxidant, vitamin C may help protect against oxidative stress and inflammation in the joints, potentially improving arthritis symptoms.

3. Vitamin E: Vitamin E is an antioxidant that may help protect against oxidative stress and inflammation in the joints, potentially improving arthritis symptoms.

4. Glucosamine and Chondroitin: These compounds are naturally found in cartilage and may help promote cartilage repair and reduce joint inflammation in osteoarthritis patients.

5. Omega-3 Fatty Acids: Omega-3 fatty acids, particularly EPA and DHA, have been shown to possess anti-inflammatory properties and may help reduce inflammation in arthritis patients.

IV Formulas for Arthritis

While IV hydration therapy is not a primary treatment for arthritis, it may help manage symptoms and support overall joint health. Some IV formulas that have been used or investigated for arthritis patients include:

1. Myers' Cocktail: A blend of vitamins and minerals, including vitamin C, magnesium, and B vitamins, which may help

address nutrient deficiencies and support overall joint health in arthritis patients.

2. High-Dose Vitamin D Infusion: High-dose vitamin D administered intravenously has been studied for its potential role in reducing inflammation and supporting immune function in arthritis patients.

3. Omega-3 Fatty Acid Infusion: IV administration of omega-3 fatty acids, particularly EPA and DHA, may help reduce inflammation in arthritis patients.

Treatment Protocol using IV Therapy

The treatment protocol for arthritis using IV therapy is highly individualized and should be tailored to the specific needs of each patient. Factors to consider include the type and severity of arthritis, nutritional status, and overall health. A possible treatment schedule might involve:

1. Myers' Cocktail: Once or twice a week for 4-6 weeks, followed by monthly maintenance infusions to support overall joint health and address nutrient deficiencies.

2. High-Dose Vitamin D Infusion: A single high-dose infusion, followed by monthly maintenance infusions if needed, depending on the patient's vitamin D levels and response to treatment.

3. Omega-3 Fatty Acid Infusion: Once or twice a month to reduce inflammation, depending on the patient's omega-3 levels and response to treatment.

References

1. Lin, J., Zhang, W., Jones, A., & Doherty, M. (2004). Efficacy of topical non-steroidal anti-inflammatory drugs in the treatment of osteoarthritis: meta-analysis of randomized controlled trials. BMJ, 329(7461), 324.

INFLAMMATORY BOWEL DISORDERS

Inflammatory bowel disorders (IBD) are a group of chronic inflammatory conditions affecting the gastrointestinal tract. The two most common forms of IBD are Crohn's disease, which can impact any part of the gastrointestinal tract, and ulcerative colitis, which affects the colon and rectum. Both conditions involve an abnormal immune response, causing inflammation and damage to the intestinal lining. IBD symptoms can include abdominal pain, diarrhea, fatigue, weight loss, and malnutrition. Management of IBD typically involves medications to reduce inflammation, surgery, and lifestyle changes to minimize symptoms.

Vitamins, Minerals, Amino Acids, and Coenzymes involved in Inflammatory Bowel Disorders

Patients with IBD often experience nutrient deficiencies due to malabsorption, inflammation, or dietary restrictions. Some key nutrients involved in managing IBD symptoms and maintaining overall health include:

1. Vitamin D: Vitamin D plays a role in immune function and may have anti-inflammatory properties. Patients with IBD

342

often have low levels of vitamin D, which can contribute to bone loss and increased susceptibility to infections.

2. Vitamin B12: Vitamin B12 is essential for red blood cell production and neurological function. Malabsorption of vitamin B12 is common in Crohn's disease patients, especially those who have had ileal resections.

3. Iron: Iron is essential for red blood cell production and oxygen transport. Iron deficiency anemia is common in IBD patients due to blood loss and inflammation-related malabsorption.

4. Zinc: Zinc is involved in immune function, wound healing, and tissue repair. Patients with IBD may have zinc deficiencies due to malabsorption, increased intestinal loss, or reduced intake.

5. Glutamine: Glutamine is an amino acid that serves as an energy source for intestinal cells and may help maintain the integrity of the intestinal barrier.

IV Formulas for Inflammatory Bowel Disorders

IV hydration therapy can help address nutrient deficiencies and dehydration in IBD patients, which may improve overall health and symptom management. Some IV formulas that have been used or investigated for IBD patients include:

1. Customized Nutrient Infusion: A tailored blend of vitamins and minerals, including vitamin D, vitamin B12, iron, and

zinc, to address individual nutrient deficiencies and support overall health.

2. Glutamine Infusion: IV administration of glutamine may help support intestinal barrier function and reduce inflammation in IBD patients.

Treatment Protocol using IV Therapy

The treatment protocol for IBD using IV therapy is highly individualized and should be tailored to the specific needs of each patient. Factors to consider include the type and severity of IBD, nutritional status, and overall health. A possible treatment schedule might involve:

1. Customized Nutrient Infusion: Once or twice a month, depending on the patient's nutrient deficiencies and response to treatment. This schedule can be adjusted based on regular monitoring of nutrient levels and symptom management.

2. Glutamine Infusion: Once or twice a week for 4-6 weeks, followed by a maintenance schedule based on the patient's response to treatment and overall health.

References

1. Garg, M., Rosella, O., Rosella, G., & Gibson, P. R. (2018). Association of circulating vitamin D concentrations with intestinal but not systemic inflammation in inflammatory bowel disease. Inflammatory Bowel Diseases, 24(3), 484-493.

2. Vagianos, K., Bector, S., & McConnell, J. (2007). Nutrition assessment of patients with inflammatory bowel disease. Journal of Parenteral and Enteral Nutrition, 31(4), 311-319.

ULCERS

Ulcers are open sores that can develop on the skin or mucous membranes. The most common type of ulcer is a peptic ulcer, which forms in the lining of the stomach, esophagus, or upper part of the small intestine. Peptic ulcers are usually caused by an imbalance between the stomach's acid production and its natural defenses, often resulting from infection with the bacterium Helicobacter pylori (H. pylori) or the use of nonsteroidal anti-inflammatory drugs (NSAIDs). Symptoms of ulcers can include abdominal pain, bloating, nausea, and weight loss. Treatment for ulcers typically involves medications to reduce stomach acid, antibiotics to treat H. pylori infections, and lifestyle changes to support healing and prevent recurrence.

Vitamins, Minerals, Amino Acids, and Coenzymes involved in Ulcers

Several nutrients play a role in the healing process of ulcers and overall gastrointestinal health. These include:

1. Vitamin C: Vitamin C is an antioxidant that helps the body produce collagen, which is essential for wound healing. Additionally, vitamin C may help eradicate H. pylori infections, a common cause of peptic ulcers.

2. Zinc: Zinc is involved in immune function, wound healing, and tissue repair. Adequate zinc levels may support ulcer

345

healing and help maintain the integrity of the gastrointestinal lining.

3. Glutamine: Glutamine is an amino acid that serves as an energy source for intestinal cells and may help maintain the integrity of the gastrointestinal lining.

4. Vitamin A: Vitamin A plays a crucial role in maintaining the integrity of the mucosal lining of the gastrointestinal tract, which may help support ulcer healing.

IV Formulas for Ulcers

While IV hydration therapy is not a primary treatment for ulcers, it can help address nutrient deficiencies and support overall gastrointestinal health. Some IV formulas that have been used or investigated for ulcers include:

1. Customized Nutrient Infusion: A tailored blend of vitamins and minerals, including vitamin C, zinc, glutamine, and vitamin A, to address individual nutrient deficiencies and support overall gastrointestinal health.

2. Glutamine Infusion: IV administration of glutamine may help support intestinal barrier function and promote healing in ulcer patients.

Treatment Protocol using IV Therapy

The treatment protocol for ulcers using IV therapy is highly individualized and should be tailored to the specific needs of each patient. Factors to consider include the type and severity of ulcers, nutritional status, and overall health. A possible treatment schedule might involve:

1. Customized Nutrient Infusion: Once or twice a month, depending on the patient's nutrient deficiencies and response to treatment. This schedule can be adjusted based on regular monitoring of nutrient levels and symptom management.

2. Glutamine Infusion: Once or twice a week for 4-6 weeks, followed by a maintenance schedule based on the patient's response to treatment and overall health.

References

1. Kato, S., Takeuchi, K., & Shimada, Y. (2001). Effect of zinc-carnosine chelate compound (Z-103), a novel antioxidant, on acute gastric mucosal injury induced by ischemia-reperfusion in rats. European Journal of Pharmacology, 427(2), 211-217.

MOOD DISORDERS

Mood disorders, also known as affective disorders, are a group of mental health conditions characterized by disturbances in mood, which can range from severe depression to extreme mania. The most common mood disorders are major depressive disorder (MDD), bipolar disorder, and persistent depressive disorder (dysthymia). The exact cause of mood disorders is not well understood, but a combination of genetic, biological, environmental, and psychological factors is believed to contribute. Treatment for mood disorders typically includes a combination of medication, psychotherapy, and lifestyle changes to help manage symptoms and improve overall well-being.

Vitamins, Minerals, Amino Acids, and Coenzymes involved in Mood Disorders

There is evidence to suggest that certain nutrients play a role in the development, progression, and treatment of mood disorders. Some of these nutrients include:

1. Vitamin D: Low levels of vitamin D have been associated with depression and mood disorders. Vitamin D is involved in various processes in the brain, including the synthesis of neurotransmitters, which are crucial for mood regulation.

2. B vitamins: B vitamins, particularly vitamin B6, B9 (folate), and B12, are essential for proper brain function and the synthesis of neurotransmitters. Deficiencies in these vitamins have been linked to mood disorders, including depression.

3. Magnesium: Magnesium is involved in many biochemical processes in the body, including those related to mood regulation. Low magnesium levels have been associated with depression and anxiety.

4. Amino acids: Amino acids such as tryptophan and tyrosine are precursors to neurotransmitters like serotonin, dopamine, and norepinephrine, which play a role in mood regulation.

IV Formulas for Mood Disorders

While IV hydration therapy is not a primary treatment for mood disorders, it can help address nutrient deficiencies and support overall mental health. Some IV formulas that have been used or investigated for mood disorders include:

1. Customized Nutrient Infusion: A tailored blend of vitamins, minerals, and amino acids, including vitamin D, B vitamins, magnesium, and amino acid precursors to neurotransmitters, to address individual nutrient deficiencies and support overall mental health.

2. Myer's Cocktail: A well-known IV formula that includes a combination of vitamins and minerals, such as B vitamins, vitamin C, magnesium, and calcium, which has been reported to improve mood and energy levels in some individuals.

Treatment Protocol using IV Therapy

The treatment protocol for mood disorders using IV therapy is highly individualized and should be tailored to the specific needs of each patient. Factors to consider include the type and severity of the mood disorder, nutritional status, and overall health. A possible treatment schedule might involve:

1. Customized Nutrient Infusion or Myer's Cocktail: Once or twice a month, depending on the patient's nutrient deficiencies and response to treatment. This schedule can be adjusted based on regular monitoring of nutrient levels and symptom management.

References

1. Anglin, R. E., Samaan, Z., Walter, S. D., & McDonald, S. D. (2013). Vitamin D deficiency and depression in adults:

systematic review and meta-analysis. The British Journal of Psychiatry, 202(2), 100-107.

2. Coppen, A., & Bolander-Gouaille, C. (2005). Treatment of depression: time to consider folic acid and vitamin B12. Journal of Psychopharmacology, 19(1), 59-65.

IMMUNOLOGICAL DISORDERS

Immunological disorders are conditions in which the immune system does not function properly. These disorders can be classified into three main categories: immunodeficiencies, autoimmune diseases, and hypersensitivity reactions. Immunodeficiencies occur when the immune system is not able to mount an adequate defense against infections and diseases. Autoimmune diseases involve the immune system attacking the body's own tissues, mistaking them for foreign invaders. Hypersensitivity reactions, such as allergies, occur when the immune system overreacts to harmless substances. Treatment for immunological disorders varies depending on the specific condition and may include medications, immunotherapy, or lifestyle changes to manage symptoms and improve overall immune function.

Vitamins, Minerals, Amino Acids, and Coenzymes involved in Immunological Disorders

Several nutrients play a role in supporting immune function and may be involved in the development or treatment of immunological disorders. These include:

1. Vitamin C: Vitamin C is a potent antioxidant and supports various cellular functions of the immune system. It is

essential for the synthesis of collagen, which is important for maintaining the integrity of tissues and organs, including the skin and blood vessels.

2. Vitamin D: Vitamin D plays a critical role in regulating immune function, and low levels have been associated with various immunological disorders, including autoimmune diseases and infections.

3. Zinc: Zinc is an essential trace element that is involved in many aspects of immune function, including cell division, gene expression, and the regulation of inflammation. Deficiency in zinc has been associated with impaired immune responses and increased susceptibility to infections.

4. Glutathione: Glutathione is a powerful antioxidant that helps maintain the balance between oxidation and reduction in cells, which is critical for proper immune function.

IV Formulas for Immunological Disorders

While IV hydration therapy is not a primary treatment for immunological disorders, it can help address nutrient deficiencies and support overall immune function. Some IV formulas that have been used or investigated for immunological disorders include:

1. Customized Nutrient Infusion: A tailored blend of vitamins, minerals, and amino acids, including vitamin C, vitamin D, zinc, and glutathione, to address individual nutrient deficiencies and support overall immune function.

2. Myer's Cocktail: A well-known IV formula that includes a combination of vitamins and minerals, such as B vitamins, vitamin C, magnesium, and calcium, which may help improve immune function and reduce inflammation.

Treatment Protocol using IV Therapy

The treatment protocol for immunological disorders using IV therapy is highly individualized and should be tailored to the specific needs of each patient. Factors to consider include the type and severity of the immunological disorder, nutritional status, and overall health. A possible treatment schedule might involve:

1. Customized Nutrient Infusion or Myer's Cocktail: Once or twice a month, depending on the patient's nutrient deficiencies and response to treatment. This schedule can be adjusted based on regular monitoring of nutrient levels and symptom management.

References

1. Carr, A. C., & Maggini, S. (2017). Vitamin C and immune function. Nutrients, 9(11), 1211.

2. Aranow, C. (2011). Vitamin D and the immune system. Journal of Investigative Medicine, 59(6), 881-886.

3. Prasad, A. S. (2008). Zinc in human health: effect of zinc on immune cells. Molecular Medicine, 14(5-6), 353-357.

MENSTRUATION

Menstruation is the natural monthly process that occurs in females of reproductive age. It involves the shedding of the uterine lining (endometrium) in response to hormonal changes if pregnancy does not occur. Menstruation typically begins during adolescence and continues until menopause. The menstrual cycle lasts approximately 28 days but can vary between individuals. Menstruation is associated with various physical and emotional symptoms, including cramps, bloating, fatigue, and mood swings. Although menstruation is a normal physiological process, some women experience severe symptoms that may require medical intervention or supportive care.

Vitamins, Minerals, Amino Acids, and Coenzymes involved in Menstruation

Several nutrients play a role in supporting overall health during menstruation and may help alleviate associated symptoms:

1. Iron: Blood loss during menstruation can lead to a decrease in iron levels, increasing the risk of anemia. Adequate iron intake is essential for maintaining healthy red blood cells and oxygen transport.

2. Vitamin B6: Vitamin B6 is involved in the production of neurotransmitters, such as serotonin and dopamine, which regulate mood. It may help alleviate mood swings and emotional symptoms related to menstruation.

3. Magnesium: Magnesium is essential for muscle and nerve function and may help reduce menstrual cramps and discomfort.

4. Calcium: Calcium is important for bone health and may help alleviate premenstrual symptoms, including mood swings, bloating, and cramping.

IV Formulas for Menstruation

While IV hydration therapy is not a primary treatment for menstruation, it can help address nutrient deficiencies and support overall health during the menstrual cycle. Some IV formulas that have been used or investigated for menstruation include:

1. Customized Nutrient Infusion: A tailored blend of vitamins, minerals, and amino acids, including iron, vitamin B6, magnesium, and calcium, to address individual nutrient deficiencies and support overall health during menstruation.

2. Myer's Cocktail: A well-known IV formula that includes a combination of vitamins and minerals, such as B vitamins, vitamin C, magnesium, and calcium, which may help improve overall health and alleviate menstrual symptoms.

Treatment Protocol using IV Therapy

The treatment protocol for menstruation using IV therapy is highly individualized and should be tailored to the specific needs of each patient. Factors to consider include the severity of menstrual symptoms, nutritional status, and overall health. A possible treatment schedule might involve:

1. Customized Nutrient Infusion or Myer's Cocktail: Once or twice a month, depending on the patient's nutrient

354

deficiencies and response to treatment. This schedule can be adjusted based on regular monitoring of nutrient levels and symptom management.

References

1. Milman, N. (2011). Iron and menstruation: facts and misconceptions. European Journal of Clinical Nutrition, 65(5), 494-499.

2. Kashanian, M., Mazinani, R., & Jalalmanesh, S. (2007). Pyridoxine (vitamin B6) therapy for premenstrual syndrome. International Journal of Gynecology & Obstetrics, 96(1), 43-44.

3. De Souza, M. C., Walker, A. F., Robinson, P. A., & Bolland, K. (2000). A synergistic effect of a daily supplement for 1 month of 200 mg magnesium plus 50 mg vitamin B6 for the relief of anxiety-related premenstrual symptoms: a randomized, double-blind, crossover study. Journal of Women's Health & Gender-Based Medicine, 9(2), 131-139.

PCOS

Polycystic ovary syndrome (PCOS) is a common hormonal disorder affecting women of reproductive age. PCOS is characterized by an imbalance of reproductive hormones, leading to the development of small cysts in the ovaries, irregular menstrual periods, and elevated levels of androgens (male hormones). This hormonal imbalance can cause various symptoms such as infertility, hirsutism (excessive hair

355

growth), acne, weight gain, and insulin resistance. PCOS is a complex condition with various contributing factors, including genetic predisposition and lifestyle choices.

Vitamins, Minerals, Amino Acids, and Coenzymes involved in PCOS

Certain nutrients play a role in supporting overall health and addressing specific symptoms or complications associated with PCOS:

1. Inositol: Inositol, a vitamin-like substance, has been shown to improve insulin sensitivity, hormone levels, and ovarian function in women with PCOS.

2. Vitamin D: Vitamin D deficiency is common in women with PCOS and may contribute to insulin resistance and hormonal imbalances.

3. Chromium: Chromium is an essential trace element that can help improve insulin sensitivity and glucose metabolism in PCOS patients.

4. Magnesium: Magnesium is involved in numerous physiological processes, including glucose metabolism, and may help improve insulin resistance in women with PCOS.

IV Formulas for PCOS

While IV hydration therapy is not a primary treatment for PCOS, it can help address nutrient deficiencies and support overall health in women with this condition. Some IV formulas that have been used or investigated for PCOS include:

1. Customized Nutrient Infusion: A tailored blend of vitamins, minerals, and amino acids, including inositol, vitamin D, chromium, and magnesium, to address individual nutrient deficiencies and support overall health in women with PCOS.

2. Myer's Cocktail: A well-known IV formula that includes a combination of vitamins and minerals, such as B vitamins, vitamin C, magnesium, and calcium, which may help improve overall health and alleviate certain PCOS symptoms.

Treatment Protocol using IV Therapy

The treatment protocol for PCOS using IV therapy is highly individualized and should be tailored to the specific needs of each patient. Factors to consider include the severity of PCOS symptoms, nutritional status, and overall health. A possible treatment schedule might involve:

1. Customized Nutrient Infusion or Myer's Cocktail: Once or twice a month, depending on the patient's nutrient deficiencies and response to treatment. This schedule can be adjusted based on regular monitoring of nutrient levels and symptom management.

References

1. Unfer, V., Nestler, J. E., Kamenov, Z. A., Prapas, N., & Facchinetti, F. (2016). Effects of Inositol(s) in Women with

PCOS: A Systematic Review of Randomized Controlled Trials. International Journal of Endocrinology, 2016, 1849162.

2. Wehr, E., Pilz, S., Schweighofer, N., Giuliani, A., Kopera, D., Pieber, T. R., & Obermayer-Pietsch, B. (2009). Association of hypovitaminosis D with metabolic disturbances in polycystic ovary syndrome. European Journal of Endocrinology, 161(4), 575-582.

INFERTILITY

Infertility is a condition characterized by the inability to conceive a child after one year of regular, unprotected intercourse. It affects both men and women and can result from various factors, including hormonal imbalances, structural abnormalities, genetic disorders, and environmental factors. Infertility can be due to problems in the female reproductive system, the male reproductive system, or a combination of both. In some cases, the cause of infertility remains unexplained.

Vitamins, Minerals, Amino Acids, and Coenzymes involved in Infertility

Certain nutrients play a role in supporting fertility by promoting reproductive health, hormonal balance, and overall wellness:

1. Folic acid: An essential B vitamin involved in DNA synthesis and cell division, crucial for the development of a healthy embryo.

2. Vitamin D: Plays a role in hormone production and regulation, and its deficiency has been linked to infertility in both men and women.

3. Coenzyme Q10 (CoQ10): An antioxidant that supports energy production in cells and may improve sperm quality and female reproductive health.

4. Omega-3 fatty acids: Essential fatty acids with anti-inflammatory properties, which may support hormonal balance and overall reproductive health.

IV Formulas for Infertility

IV hydration therapy is not a primary treatment for infertility, but it can help address nutrient deficiencies and support overall health in individuals trying to conceive. Some IV formulas that have been used or investigated for infertility include:

1. Customized Nutrient Infusion: A tailored blend of vitamins, minerals, and amino acids, including folic acid, vitamin D, CoQ10, and omega-3 fatty acids, to address individual nutrient deficiencies and support fertility.

2. Myer's Cocktail: A well-known IV formula that includes a combination of vitamins and minerals, such as B vitamins, vitamin C, magnesium, and calcium, which may help improve overall health and support fertility.

Treatment Protocol using IV Therapy

The treatment protocol for infertility using IV therapy is highly individualized and should be tailored to the specific needs of each patient. Factors to consider include the severity of infertility, nutritional status, and overall health. A possible treatment schedule might involve:

1. Customized Nutrient Infusion or Myer's Cocktail: Once or twice a month, depending on the patient's nutrient deficiencies and response to treatment. This schedule can be adjusted based on regular monitoring of nutrient levels and overall reproductive health.

References

1. Gaskins, A. J., Chiu, Y. H., Williams, P. L., Ford, J. B., Toth, T. L., Hauser, R., & Chavarro, J. E. (2016). Association between serum folate and vitamin B-12 and outcomes of assisted reproductive technologies. The American Journal of Clinical Nutrition, 104(4), 997-1004.

2. Lerchbaum, E., & Obermayer-Pietsch, B. (2012). Vitamin D and fertility: a systematic review. European Journal of Endocrinology, 166(5), 765-778.

3. Safarinejad, M. R., Safarinejad, S., & Shafiei, N. (2012). Effects of the reduced form of coenzyme Q10 (ubiquinol) on semen parameters in men with idiopathic infertility: a double-blind, placebo-controlled, randomized study. Journal of Urology, 188(2), 526-531.

PREOPERATIVE PERIOD

The pre-surgical period, also known as the preoperative period, refers to the time leading up to a surgical procedure. During this period, patients are typically assessed for their overall health, medical history, and potential risks associated with the surgery. The pre-surgical period is important for optimizing patient health and ensuring that they are in the best possible condition for surgery, which can help improve surgical outcomes and minimize complications.

Vitamins, Minerals, Amino Acids, and Coenzymes involved in Pre-Surgical Preparation

Certain nutrients can play a crucial role in preparing the body for surgery by supporting immune function, wound healing, and overall well-being:

1. Vitamin C: Essential for collagen synthesis, tissue repair, and immune function.

2. Vitamin A: Supports epithelial cell growth, wound healing, and immune function.

3. B Vitamins: Important for energy production, immune function, and tissue repair.

4. Zinc: Plays a role in protein synthesis, cell division, and wound healing.

5. Glutamine: An amino acid involved in immune function and intestinal health, which may be depleted during surgery and stress.

6. Arginine: An amino acid that supports wound healing and immune function.

IV Formulas for Pre-Operative Healing and Infection Prevention

IV hydration therapy can help pre-surgical patients by providing essential nutrients to optimize their health and support their immune function. Some commonly used IV formulas include:

1. Myer's Cocktail: A well-known IV formula containing a blend of vitamins and minerals, such as B vitamins, vitamin C, magnesium, and calcium, which may help support overall health and recovery.

2. Immune Boost Infusion: A customized IV formula containing nutrients that specifically support immune function and wound healing, such as vitamin C, vitamin A, zinc, glutamine, and arginine.

Treatment Protocol using IV Therapy

The treatment protocol for IV therapy in pre-surgical patients should be tailored to individual needs and may vary depending on factors such as the type of surgery, patient's overall health, and nutritional status. A possible treatment schedule could involve:

1. Myer's Cocktail or Immune Boost Infusion: Administered 1-2 weeks prior to surgery, followed by additional infusions as needed, based on the patient's response to treatment and surgical team recommendations.

References

1. Engelman, D. T., Ben Ali, W., Williams, J. B., Perrault, L. P., Reddy, V. S., Arora, R. C., ... & Lamy, A. (2012). Guidelines

for perioperative care in cardiac surgery: Enhanced Recovery After Surgery Society recommendations. JAMA Surgery, 154(8), 755-766.

2. Ljungqvist, O., Scott, M., & Fearon, K. C. (2017). Enhanced Recovery After Surgery: A review. JAMA Surgery, 152(3), 292-298.

3. Gouin, J. P., Kiecolt-Glaser, J. K., Malarkey, W. B., & Glaser, R. (2008). The influence of anger expression on wound healing. Brain, Behavior, and Immunity, 22(5), 699-708.

4. Mora, J. R., Iwata, M., & von Andrian, U. H. (2008). Vitamin effects on the immune system: vitamins A and D take centre stage. Nature Reviews Immunology, 8(9), 685-698.

POSTOPERATIVE PERIOD

The post-surgical period, also known as the postoperative period, refers to the time following a surgical procedure. This period is critical for patient recovery and typically involves monitoring vital signs, managing pain, preventing complications, and promoting healing. The duration of the post-surgical period varies depending on the type of surgery, the patient's overall health, and the presence of any complications.

Vitamins, Minerals, Amino Acids, and Coenzymes involved in Post-Surgical Recovery

During post-surgical recovery, certain nutrients play a crucial role in supporting the healing process, immune function, and overall well-being:

1. Vitamin C: Essential for collagen synthesis and tissue repair, as well as immune function.

2. Vitamin A: Supports epithelial cell growth, wound healing, and immune function.

3. B Vitamins: Important for energy production, immune function, and tissue repair.

4. Zinc: Plays a role in protein synthesis, cell division, and wound healing.

5. Glutamine: An amino acid involved in immune function and intestinal health, which may be depleted during surgery and stress.

6. Arginine: An amino acid that supports wound healing and immune function.

IV Formulas for Post-Operative Healing and Infection Prevention

IV hydration therapy can help post-surgical patients by providing essential nutrients for recovery and supporting immune function. Some commonly used IV formulas include:

1. Myer's Cocktail: A well-known IV formula containing a blend of vitamins and minerals, such as B vitamins, vitamin C, magnesium, and calcium, which may help support overall health and recovery.

2. Immune Boost Infusion: A customized IV formula containing nutrients that specifically support immune function and

wound healing, such as vitamin C, vitamin A, zinc, glutamine, and arginine.

Treatment Protocol using IV Therapy

The treatment protocol for IV therapy in post-surgical patients should be tailored to individual needs and may vary depending on factors such as the type of surgery, patient's overall health, and nutritional status. A possible treatment schedule could involve:

1. Myer's Cocktail or Immune Boost Infusion: Administered within 24-48 hours post-surgery, followed by additional infusions as needed, based on the patient's recovery progress and response to treatment.

References

1. Blass, S. C., Goost, H., Tolba, R. H., Stoffel-Wagner, B., Kabir, K., Burger, C., ... & Stehle, P. (2012). Time to wound closure in trauma patients with disorders in wound healing is shortened by supplements containing antioxidant micronutrients and glutamine: a PRCT. Clinical Nutrition, 31(4), 469-475.

2. Braga, M., Gianotti, L., Nespoli, L., Radaelli, G., & Di Carlo, V. (2002). Nutritional approach in malnourished surgical patients: a prospective randomized study. Archives of Surgery, 137(2), 174-180.

3. Delmi, M., Rapin, C. H., Bengoa, J. M., Delmas, P. D., Vasey, H., & Bonjour, J. P. (1990). Dietary supplementation in

elderly patients with fractured neck of the femur. The Lancet, 335(8696), 1013-1016.

CONCLUSION

IV Hydration clinics are in high demand. But at the same time the rise in IV hydration clinics is also high. In order to differentiate yourself, it's important to niche into an area.

In this book, we have compiled a comprehensive overview of vitamins, minerals, amino acids, enzymes and peptides that are used in IV Hydration. This is not an exhaustive list, but it's robust. Any clinic owner should be able to find an area to specialize in - whether it's IV hydration for a particular condition or a particular drip.

We encourage you to use this book as foundational knowledge. Formulas are largely concocted at the individual clinic level. There is no consensus on the right amount, the right frequency, the right duration.

We have provided some solid guidelines that can start you off on a productive conversation with your medical director and pharmacist to create your own protocols.

Research is constant and new elements are being found, promoted or rediscovered. Keep on top of this research on an ongoing basis for yourself and for your clients.

APPENDIX - 797 GUIDELINES

The US Pharmacopeia (USP) General Chapter 797 provides guidelines for the safe compounding of sterile preparations, including intravenous (IV) therapy. These guidelines were developed to help prevent contamination and ensure the safety and efficacy of compounded sterile preparations, including IV medications.

The USP Chapter 797 guidelines cover a wide range of topics related to IV therapy, including:

1. Facilities and equipment: This includes requirements for the design and construction of clean rooms and other compounding areas, as well as specifications for equipment such as laminar flow hoods and biological safety cabinets.

    a. Clean room or compounding area: A clean room or compounding area is a designated area where sterile preparations are compounded. It should be constructed to meet specific design and environmental requirements, including positive air pressure, controlled temperature, and humidity, as well as proper air filtration and circulation. The clean room should be separated from other areas in the facility to prevent cross-contamination.

    b. Laminar flow hood: A laminar flow hood is a piece of equipment that provides a sterile environment for compounding. It uses HEPA (high-efficiency particulate air) filters to filter air entering the hood, and a vertical airflow to create a sterile work environment. A laminar flow hood is used for compounding low and medium-risk sterile preparations.

c. Biological safety cabinet: A biological safety cabinet (BSC) is similar to a laminar flow hood but provides additional protection for the compounder and the environment. A BSC provides a physical barrier between the compounding area and the operator, and uses HEPA filters to filter air entering and exiting the cabinet. A BSC is used for compounding high-risk sterile preparations and hazardous drugs.

d. Equipment and supplies: Various equipment and supplies are required for sterile compounding, including vials, syringes, needles, filters, gowns, gloves, and disinfectants. All equipment and supplies should be sterile and non-toxic.

e. Environmental monitoring equipment: Environmental monitoring equipment is used to monitor the air quality in the compounding area, including particle counts, temperature, humidity, and pressure differentials. Environmental monitoring helps to ensure that the compounding area meets the required standards for cleanliness and air quality.

2. Personnel training and qualifications: The guidelines outline the training and qualifications required for personnel involved in compounding sterile preparations, including IV medications.

    a. Education and training: Personnel involved in sterile compounding should have appropriate education and training in compounding sterile preparations, including IV medications. They should also be knowledgeable about relevant regulations, standards, and guidelines.

    b. Competency assessment: Personnel should be assessed for their knowledge, skills, and abilities related to sterile compounding. Competency assessments may include written and practical tests, as well as ongoing performance evaluations.

    c. Aseptic technique: Personnel should be trained in aseptic technique, which involves preventing the introduction of microorganisms into sterile preparations. Aseptic technique training should include proper hand hygiene, gowning, gloving, and disinfection procedures.

    d. Personal protective equipment: Personnel should be trained in the proper use of personal protective equipment, including gowns, gloves, masks, and eye protection. They should also be trained in the proper disposal of contaminated materials.

e. Continuing education: Personnel should receive ongoing education and training to stay up-to-date with the latest standards and guidelines for sterile compounding.

f. Supervision: Personnel involved in sterile compounding should be supervised by qualified personnel with appropriate knowledge and training in sterile compounding.

g. Classroom instruction: Classroom instruction provides a foundation of knowledge on aseptic technique, sterile compounding, and the compounding process. This may include courses on microbiology, pharmacology, and USP General Chapter 797.

h. Hands-on training: Hands-on training is critical to the development of the skills required for the preparation of CSPs. This may include training on the use of sterile compounding equipment, such as laminar flow hoods and syringe pumps, and sterile techniques, such as hand hygiene and gowning.

i. Competency assessment: Competency assessment is an important component of training to ensure that personnel have the knowledge and skills necessary to perform their job functions. This may include written tests, practical assessments, and ongoing evaluations of performance.

j. Continuing education: Continuing education is necessary to ensure that personnel stay up-to-date with the latest developments in aseptic technique, sterile compounding, and the compounding process. This may include attending conferences, workshops, and seminars, as well as online courses and webinars.

k. Refresher training: Refresher training is important to reinforce the knowledge and skills learned during initial training and to ensure that personnel remain competent. Refresher training may be required on a periodic basis, such as annually or bi-annually.

3. Environmental monitoring: This involves regularly testing the air and surfaces in clean rooms and other compounding areas to ensure that they are free from contaminants.

a. Particle counts: Environmental monitoring includes the measurement of airborne particles in the compounding area, using a laser particle counter. The particle count is used to determine the level of cleanliness of the compounding area and to ensure that it meets the required standards.

b. Surface sampling: Environmental monitoring includes the collection of samples from surfaces in the compounding area, using a swab or contact plate. Surface sampling is used to identify potential sources of contamination and to assess the effectiveness of cleaning procedures.

c. Microbial testing: Environmental monitoring may include the testing of samples for microbial contamination, using culture-based methods or molecular methods. Microbial testing is used to identify potential sources of contamination and to assess the effectiveness of disinfection procedures.

d. Temperature, humidity, and pressure: Environmental monitoring includes the measurement of temperature, humidity, and pressure in the compounding area, using sensors. These parameters are important for maintaining a stable and controlled environment for sterile compounding.

e. Record-keeping: Environmental monitoring data should be recorded and maintained for a specified period, as per the facility's policy. The data should be reviewed regularly to identify trends and to ensure that the compounding area meets the required standards.

4. Cleaning and disinfection: The guidelines specify the procedures and agents that should be used to clean and disinfect compounding areas and equipment.

5. Compounding procedures: The guidelines provide detailed instructions for the preparation of sterile compounded preparations, including IV medications, and the handling of hazardous drugs.

a. Gather supplies: Collect all the necessary supplies, including the medication vial, sterile syringe and needle, sterile gloves, alcohol swabs, and a sterile vial adapter.

b. Wash hands and don personal protective equipment: Perform proper hand hygiene and put on appropriate personal protective equipment, including a sterile gown, gloves, mask, and eye protection.

c. Clean work area: Clean the work area with a disinfectant solution and allow it to air dry.

d. Verify medication order: Verify the medication order against the patient's medical record and the medication label.

e. Prepare the medication: Use aseptic technique to prepare the medication by adding the appropriate amount of diluent to the vial, if necessary. Withdraw the correct amount of medication into the sterile syringe.

f. Attach the vial adapter: Attach the sterile vial adapter to the medication vial, ensuring that it is firmly in place.

g. Mix the medication: Use a gentle swirling motion to mix the medication thoroughly.

h. Attach the syringe: Attach the sterile syringe to the vial adapter and slowly inject the medication into the vial.

i. Remove the syringe: Remove the syringe and vial adapter from the vial.

j. Label the syringe: Label the syringe with the patient's name, medication name and strength, dose, and expiration date.

k. Clean the work area: Clean the work area with a disinfectant solution and allow it to air dry.

l. Administer the medication: Administer the medication via the appropriate IV route, according to facility policy.

m. Dispose of supplies: Dispose of all used supplies in the appropriate containers.

6. Quality control and assurance: This includes testing of compounded preparations to ensure their sterility and potency, as well as monitoring of compounding processes to identify and correct any issues that may arise.

7. Overall, the USP Chapter 797 guidelines are designed to help ensure the safety and quality of IV therapy and other sterile compounding practices. It is important for healthcare providers and facilities to follow these guidelines to prevent adverse events and ensure positive patient outcomes.

It is important for facilities and healthcare providers to follow these requirements for facilities and equipment to ensure that sterile preparations, including IV medications, are compounded safely and effectively. Regular maintenance and testing of equipment and facilities are also important to ensure ongoing compliance with 797 guidelines.

The USP General Chapter 797 defines Low-Risk level CSPs as:

- Simple aseptic transfer of sterile drug or nutrients into sterile containers

- Reconstitution of sterile drug or nutrients using aseptic technique

- Preparation of sterile products using only sterile ingredients and devices that are all terminally sterilized before use

- Preparation of sterile products using only sterile, non-hazardous, and non-radioactive ingredients and devices that are all terminally sterilized before use

Examples of Low-Risk level CSPs include:

- Preparation of a single dose of a medication for immediate use

- Reconstitution of a single dose of a medication using aseptic technique

- Preparation of total parenteral nutrition (TPN) solutions using pre-mixed, sterile components

- Low-Risk level CSPs can be prepared in a cleanroom or in a segregated area that meets the requirements for a low-risk level CSP. These requirements include:

- Aseptic technique and proper hand hygiene

- Use of sterile, single-use devices

- Cleaning and disinfecting of the preparation area and equipment

- Environmental monitoring to ensure air quality and surface cleanliness

- Labeling of the CSP with the medication name, strength, dose, and beyond-use date.

If you're interested in owning an IV hydration business, it's essential to understand the US Pharmacopeia (USP) General Chapter 797 guidelines for sterile compounding of IV preparations. These guidelines were developed to prevent contamination and ensure the safety and efficacy of compounded sterile preparations, including IV medications.

The guidelines cover a wide range of topics, including facility design and equipment requirements, personnel training and qualifications, and environmental monitoring. Below are some guidelines to consider when starting an IV hydration business:

Facilities and Equipment:

You need a clean room or compounding area where sterile preparations are compounded. The area should meet specific design and environmental requirements, including positive air pressure, controlled temperature, and humidity, as well as proper air filtration and circulation. It should be separated from other areas in the facility to prevent cross-contamination. You will also need laminar flow hoods and biological safety cabinets to create a sterile environment.

Equipment and Supplies:

Various equipment and supplies are required for sterile compounding, including vials, syringes, needles, filters, gowns, gloves, and disinfectants. All equipment and supplies should be sterile and non-toxic.

Personnel Training and Qualifications:

Personnel involved in sterile compounding should have appropriate education and training in compounding sterile preparations, including IV medications. They should also be knowledgeable about relevant regulations, standards, and guidelines. Personnel should be trained in aseptic technique, including proper hand hygiene, gowning, gloving, and disinfection procedures. They should also be trained in the proper use and disposal of personal protective equipment.

Continuing Education:

Personnel should receive ongoing education and training to stay up-to-date with the latest standards and guidelines for sterile compounding. Continuing education may include attending conferences, workshops, and seminars, as well as online courses and webinars. Refresher training is important to reinforce the knowledge and skills learned during initial training and to ensure that personnel remain competent.

Environmental Monitoring:

Regularly testing the air and surfaces in clean rooms and other compounding areas is crucial to ensure that they are free from contaminants. Environmental monitoring includes measuring airborne particles, collecting samples from surfaces in the compounding area, and testing samples for microbial contamination. Monitoring the temperature, humidity, and pressure is also essential.

In conclusion, the USP General Chapter 797 guidelines for sterile compounding of IV medications are essential to ensure patient safety and prevent contamination. To own an IV hydration business, you must follow these guidelines and ensure that your facility and personnel are properly trained and qualified.

There are services that provide environmental monitoring for IV hydration clinics. These services typically test for a range of environmental factors, such as air quality, temperature, humidity, and water quality. The frequency of monitoring may vary depending on local regulations, but it is generally recommended that monitoring be done at least annually, if not more frequently.

It's important for IV hydration clinics to ensure that their facilities are clean and free from any environmental hazards that could compromise patient safety. Regular monitoring can help identify any potential issues and allow for timely corrective action to be taken. It's best to consult with a qualified environmental monitoring service provider to determine the appropriate monitoring schedule for your particular clinic.

Made in the USA
Middletown, DE
23 May 2025